Making
the
BREAST
of It

Robin Storey

Making the BREAST of It

Breast Cancer Stories of Humour and Joy

Cover design by Custom E-Book Covers
www.customebookcovers.com

Copyediting by Christine's Edits
www.christinesedits.com

Interior layout by Maureen Cutajar
www.gopublished.com

To my family
For all your love and support
before, during and after my treatment

Introduction

'What humour and joy is there in breast cancer?' You may well be asking.

Perhaps you're still in the first throes of shock after a diagnosis that has shaken the foundations of your world. Or bald, haggard and exhausted after another round of chemotherapy, or coming to terms with losing a 'bosom' buddy. Or both. Or you may be lucky, like me—stage 1 breast cancer—lumpectomy, radiation therapy and medication.

Every woman's experience of breast cancer is different, and I'm not by any means minimising the trauma of it. Whatever your diagnosis, you can count on tears; depression; dark fears that ambush you in the middle of the night; snapping at your spouse and/or kids because you're feeling crappy; and having a meltdown when the printer jams. All perfectly normal.

But it's also important to laugh and find joy because it will help to heal you just as much as your medication. There's a ton of research indicating that laughter has many healing properties and can play a big role in your recovery. And joy is everywhere when you start looking for it. It may show up you when you least expect it, so you find yourself giggling to yourself in the doctor's

1

waiting room or your heart bursting with bliss as you stroll along a secluded beach.

In this book I share my own experiences and those of other breast cancer survivors from all walks of life. Some I have met in person during the course of my journey; others I've discovered on the internet. I got to know a bunch of courageous women— Rochelle, Katie, Jan, Yvonne and Kath—whose thoughts and experiences I've included in this book, as well as my close friend Kay, whom I'm known since school. Their surnames have been withheld for privacy.

Amongst us all, I think we've provided enough material for any self-respecting stand-up comedian, and I hope this book brings you joy, and lots of laughs.

The Phone Call

I'm at work when I receive a message on my mobile phone to ring Sharon from BreastScreen. I know instantly this can't be good. They've never called me—my mammograms, which I've had religiously every two years since I turned 40, have always been clear. I had one just a couple of weeks ago. I call the number; but it goes to an answering machine, so I leave a message. But when Sharon hasn't returned my call in ten minutes, I phone again. If it's bad news, I want to know now.

'The results of your mammogram have shown there's something in your left breast the doctors want to have a closer look at,' Sharon says. 'Can you come in for some further tests?'

We make an appointment for three days time. I'm in the office by myself and tears are streaming down my face. I can't die now, not before I have grandchildren! I want to cuddle them and take them to the park, and tell them stories and spoil them rotten. And what about my children? They'll be devastated—I can't bear to die and make them so sad.

It's funny how the mind processes shock. I go straight from 'there's something in your left breast' to death. Although my three children are all adults, I'm a long way off being a grandmother,

3

and I'm quite content for them to produce offspring when they're ready.

But my non-existent grandchildren are the first things that spring to mind. And never mind that it might be sad for me to die—I don't want to be the cause of my children's sadness by being so inconsiderate as to die.

I immediately email my partner Aaron. 'Oh, crap' is his empathetic reply. I'm so glad he didn't come up with the usual platitude of 'I'm sure it will be fine'. Because I know in my gut there's a chance it won't be.

Many breast cancer survivors I've spoken to had a similar experience when first told there was something wrong, even before diagnosis.

'You immediately think of death.'

'My first thought was, "How will my husband cope without me?"'

'I burst into tears and wailed, "I'm not ready to die!"'

Thinking back on it now, I try to analyse that reaction. Despite the modern advances in treatment for cancer and the fact that many people make a complete recovery from it, cancer is still a word that evokes a lot of emotion. Usually fear. Because we all know someone, or of someone, who has died from cancer. And for every story we hear of a cancer survivor, there's another story of someone who lost the battle.

It's also our fear of uncertainty that comes into play. Cancer often strikes without warning. It doesn't care how old you are and whether you've lived a life of purity and wholesomeness, not allowing even a square of chocolate to pass your lips or a cyclone to interfere with your marathon training. Anyone is fair game. Which is brought home to us with startling clarity when we get that phone call or letter.

Or maybe immediately thinking the worst is our subconscious protecting us, so we're prepared for it if it happens. If it doesn't, all the more cause for celebration.

Enough of the psychoanalysing – you could twist yourself in

knots thinking about it. After the initial shock has subsided, I give myself a severe talking to. 'Of course you're not going to die, you don't even know if it *is* cancer.'

It's hard to concentrate on my work for the rest of the day. What did she mean by 'something' in my left breast? Is it a spot, a lump or a nebulous mass? Or a euphemism for 'Get her in straight away before it's too late?'

At home that night, I check in with Dr Google. According to it, 90% of mammogram callbacks are clear. So the odds are in my favour. That cheers me up considerably, especially after I talk on the phone with my close friend Kay.

At 60, Kay is a few months older than me. She was first diagnosed with breast cancer at 40. After treatment and 15 years in the clear, the cancer came back in the same breast. After another round of treatment, it resurfaced a third time; so finally acknowledging that her breast was out to get her, she had a mastectomy and breast reconstruction. She then had a reduction on her other breast to ensure she had a matching pair.

She got through it all with such quiet courage and humour that I call her 'The Poster Girl for Breast Cancer'. There should be posters of her in bus shelters, in a tight sweater showing off her new perky boobs and with the exhortation, 'You, too, can survive breast cancer! Make an appointment for a mammogram today!'

Kay agrees there's a good chance my tests will be clear. 'And even if you do have cancer, you'll get the best treatment. The specialists are absolutely fantastic.'

I'm almost convinced.

A Testing Time

The rain is coming down hard and fast. The BreastScreen clinic I have to attend is behind the local hospital, and the underground car park is already full at 8.30 am. The only car park I can get is about three blocks away, at a roadside parking bay that clearly states it's three hour-parking.

Sharon told me to expect to be there for four hours at the most—I'm hoping it won't be that long as parking inspectors regularly patrol this road. I've come prepared with a book and an apple. Aaron has offered to come with me but I've told him there's no need. They're only tests.

When I arrive and am checked in by the receptionist, I'm taken to a change room where I take off my bra and top, and put on a hospital gown. I'm then directed to a waiting room where lots of women about my age and older are sitting around in hospital gowns, chatting away as if they've known each other all their lives.

I open my book and start reading. A friendly middle-aged volunteer named Joy (according to her lanyard) is doing the rounds and chatting to everyone. I'm not in the mood for small talk, but I make polite conversation when it's my turn.

7

After a while, a nurse calls me in, explains the various tests I may undergo and I sign a consent form. I'm called in again to have an ultrasound then I return to the waiting room before my interview with the doctor. A steady parade of previous occupants passes through, giving whoops of joy and clutching their bits of paper—their passports to a cancer-free future—on their way to the dressing rooms to get changed. Some of them give Joy a hug.

I'm still sitting there. I have this absurd feeling that they've all passed an exam, which I've failed. I have to stay behind and see the doctor as punishment. The niggle that's been in my stomach since I've walked in becomes a horrible certainty. I didn't make it into the 90 percenters.

Eventually I'm called in. The doctor explains that the scan has confirmed the presence of a lump in my left breast. She gets me up on the bed, prods the lower half of my left breast and says, 'There it is.'

She guides my hand to it and I feel it, like a small hard pea. Just as I've heard it described so many times by women who've had breast cancer.

'The best procedure now would be a core biopsy to determine the nature of the lump,' she says. 'Are you okay with that?'

I nod numbly. She's talking about further courses of action—radiation and chemotherapy.

'But of course,' she says, 'it may be benign.'

Why do I get the feeling she doesn't really believe that?

I'm ushered into the treatment room again where I greet the sonographer who did my ultrasound like an old friend. She gels up my good breast and gives it the once-over. God forbid I I should have a lump in the other breast! Fortunately, it's clear.

The biopsy is over in a few minutes with one of the nurses, Jodie, holding my hand throughout the procedure. It's not painful as I've been given a local anaesthetic, but not pleasant either.

'Would you like to see what we took out?' the doctor asks.

I almost gag at the thought.

'No thanks,' I say hastily. Is it common practice these days for doctors to offer to let you view pieces of your body they've removed?

'Would you like to look at this nasty carbuncle we've just removed? Don't mind all the blood and pus.'

'Take a gander at your gall bladder—what a beauty!'

I'm then sent back to the waiting room again with an ice pack pressed to my breast inside my hospital gown. The waiting room is almost empty. I feel even more like the kid who's had to stay behind after school. The nurse calls me in to the dressing room, gives me some post-op instructions and makes another appointment for Wednesday to get the results of the biopsy. Four days away.

I was in there for well over three hours; and as I trudge back to my car in the rain, I think to myself, 'Now all I need is a parking ticket.'

The more I think about it, the more incensed I become. How dare that parking inspector take advantage of someone in such a vulnerable state, who may very well have cancer! I could hardly go dashing up the street in my hospital gown, ice pack pressed to one boob and the other threatening to pop out at any minute, to move my car.

I'll fight this. I'll take legal action. I can see the headlines in the local paper. Breast Cancer Patient Takes Council to Court over Parking Fine. Accompanied by a photo of me smiling with brave determination—the spokesperson for all downtrodden patients (the victims of 'manifestly inadequate parking facilities' at the hospital).

When I get to the car, there's no parking ticket on the windscreen getting sodden in the rain. Thank God for wimpy parking inspectors who don't want to get wet.

The Waiting

I lead a busy life so the time goes quickly, but at the same time excruciatingly slowly. I've told Aaron of course, some of my family (but not my children as I don't want to worry them unnecessarily in case the results are clear) and a couple of close friends.

'Think positively,' says one friend. As if that's going to make any difference.

'It won't be cancer,' Aaron says with all the confidence of someone who's not going through it. Waiting for test results is one of the hardest things to do; and in clinical studies, breast cancer patients have reported that awaiting the results of their initial biopsy is the most distressing part of the whole cancer experience.

From my own experience, I agree wholeheartedly. I'm very aware that these results have the potential to drastically change the course of my life. And little do I know at this stage that in the months ahead, I'll become an expert on waiting for test results.

I read all sorts of advice on the internet about how to cope with the waiting period—exercise, meditation, time out with friends and family and distracting yourself with activities.

I do all of those things, with limited success. I try not to think about it as I know that being anxious is pointless and a waste of energy. But my mind keeps coming back to it when it thinks I'm not looking; like a naughty kid constantly going to the cookie jar.

It conjures up scenes of pathos worthy of a Hollywood tear-jerker—me gathering my children around me and breaking the news to them, sitting up in my hospital bed after my operation, pale and wan, shaving my head before chemo so I don't have to put up with my hair falling out. I've often wondered if I could carry off the bald look, but now would be more than happy to keep wondering. Tears spring unbidden to my eyes even when I'm not consciously thinking about cancer.

On the weekend, Aaron and I go for a hike in Noosa National Park, a scenic walk that skirts the coastline. It's a glorious day—dazzling blue sky and glittering waves—and I really try to anchor myself in the present and enjoy my surroundings. But at the end of the walk I'm exhausted from wrestling my mind away from thinking about cancer and guilty that I haven't enjoyed it as much as I'd hoped. I feel much better after coffee and cake – sugar and caffeine was what I needed, not communing with nature.

One of the things that worries me most is that Aaron and I had planned to leave in three weeks for a four-week overseas trip. If the test results are positive, will we have to cancel the trip so I can have treatment? We're booked into a three-day conference on internet marketing in San Diego, and the rest of the trip is sightseeing around California. We've both been very excited about it and will be devastated if we can't go. We still have a couple of day trips to book but we hold off. My life is in limbo.

On Monday night, I decide on impulse to write down all the thoughts and feelings I've had since the first phone call from BreastScreen. I have an online journal that's been very neglected, so I log in and start writing. It all comes pouring out; and when I've finished, I feel ten tons lighter. What a revelation! I'm so glad it only took me three days to work out that as a writer I would find solace in writing.

The night before my appointment to get my test results, I write in my diary:

'Tomorrow is D (Diagnosis) Day. After wishing it would hurry up and arrive, now I don't want to know. The uncertainty that has been so tortuous up to this point now seems preferable to knowing the truth. Breast cancer is like a foreign country that I've heard a lot about but have no desire to go to. The inhabitants seem like a warm and friendly lot, not to mention courageous, but I don't want to be one of them.'

The Results

Aaron and I are sitting in the waiting room of the Breast-Screen clinic. 'I'm not going to cry,' I tell myself firmly. 'I'll hold it all together.'

The doctor, a young woman, calls us in. Jodie, the nurse who held my hand during the biopsy, follows us in. This confirms what I have known deep in my subconscious all week. You don't need a doctor and a nurse to tell you your test is clear.

'The test has confirmed that there's cancer,' the doctor says. I immediately burst into tears. Jodie hands me a box of tissues. They must get bulk orders of these.

I try to concentrate on what the doctor is telling me. The lump is small; there's no indication that the cancer has spread, or that I will need a mastectomy or chemotherapy. Although they won't know for sure until after surgery, it seems that removal of the lump (a lumpectomy) and six weeks of radiation therapy is all the treatment I'll need. The best possible result under the circumstances.

After the shock of hearing the word 'cancer', my next thought is, 'Can we still go on our overseas trip?' The other good news is that we can. The cancer is not aggressive and surgery can be scheduled for after our return. Jodie gives me a ton of resources from the Cancer Council to take home—a folder full of information about breast cancer and a list of support agencies, a book about early breast cancer, another on how to cope with a cancer diagnosis, a relaxation CD and another for partners on how to support someone with breast cancer.

There's nothing more to do now except wait for the letter informing me of my surgery date. As soon as Aaron and I get out the front door of the clinic, I burst into tears again. And so does he. It's one of the few times I've seen him cry.

We sit on a nearby bench seat for a while. I bet it's been privy to a flood of tears. It's probably why it was put there. There should be a plaque on it. The Crying Seat.

'You'd better not die,' Aaron warns.

'Of course I'm not going to die,' I sniffle.

On the drive home, I reflect that contrary to my thoughts of the previous night, knowledge is better than uncertainty. Knowledge means I can take action.

People react in all sorts of ways to the news of a cancer diagnosis—shock, disbelief, anger and every emotion in between. Often the shock leaves you numb and the other emotions come flooding in later. One thing is common to everyone: like your memory of finding out about the assassination of John Lennon or 9/11, you never forget that moment, frozen forever in time, when you find out you have breast cancer.

Kay only had a mammogram to appease a friend who insisted she go because a friend of his had just been diagnosed with breast cancer. At 40, it was her first mammogram.

'I was in total shock—and denial. I just didn't want to know.' Shortly after her diagnosis, a friend took her to a breast cancer information session, but she walked out soon after it started because she didn't want to hear it.

'The first thing you think of is death,' says Jan. 'Your whole body drains; your head goes fuzzy—you just can't think.'

Kath was a nurse working with AIDS patients when told of

her diagnosis. 'My first thought was, "So this is what it's like to be told you might die."'

Florence Strang, co-author of the book *100 Perks of Having Cancer plus 100 Health Tips For Surviving It,* was the eternal optimist when told she had Stage 3 breast cancer. 'My first thought was Stage 3. That means 3 out of 10. That's not so bad. At least I'm still in the early stages. Then I discovered that Stage 4 is as bad as it gets. I had some serious cancer to deal with!'

Whatever your initial reaction to your diagnosis, it takes some time for it to sink in and for you to process the news.

Breaking The News

By the time I get home, I've pulled myself together sufficiently to ring family and close friends with the news. 'I have breast cancer,' I tell them, but it doesn't feel real. I may as well be saying, 'I have turned into a werewolf.' I am now an inhabitant of that foreign country called Breast Cancer, but I still feel like a stranger.

I manage to get through all the conversations without breaking down. Apart from the fact that I'm uncomfortable crying in front of other people, even those close to me, I feel the need to put up a brave front; so they'll know I'm okay and won't worry about me.

My three children, ranging in age from 30 to 24, are the ones whose reactions I'm most concerned about. One of my daughters, Cassie, has been living in Canada for the last four years— my other daughter Emma and son Tim live in Brisbane, 100 kilometres away,

I email them initially so they all have the same information at the same time, and because I'm afraid I won't be able to recount the facts once, let alone three times, without bursting into tears. Telling my children I have cancer is a very different proposition

19

to that of telling others, and I find it the most emotionally wrenching part of the breaking-the-news process. I think about how I would have felt if my own mother had been diagnosed with cancer: shock (other people's mothers get cancer, not mine!), anxiety, panic and fear of losing her.

After they've had a chance to read the email, I phone each of the children to expound on my initial information and answer any questions they might have. I make it clear I'm not going to die. They're naturally shocked and concerned; and it's especially hard for Cassie, hearing the news and being so far from home. But they seem reassured by my assurances and that's a big relief.

Thank goodness the next two days are my rostered days off work as I only work part-time. I had a list of things planned, but I spend a lot of the time sitting on the couch in tears. I email my supervisor at work with the news. I have three months sick leave up my sleeve and have decided that I will commence it as soon as I get back from my holidays. I expect my lumpectomy to be fairly soon after my return.

He emails back and says that he knows I've been under a lot of stress at work, implying that it could be a contributing factor in my getting cancer. It's true that my job as a probation and parole officer is stressful and has become more so in the last couple of years—even though I only work three days a week. Is this a sign that I should find another way to earn a living?

It's Mother's Day four days after diagnosis, and Emma and Tim arrive the night before. My brother joins us and we have a roast dinner, and then play Cards Against Humanity and Uno Attack. Both games have become favourites with our family and are guaranteed to produce much hilarity, especially when accompanied by the consumption of alcohol. There's no greater therapy than laughter and family togetherness.

The next morning is a glorious autumn day. The sun is high in the sky and the world is bright. We go to a new cafe, The Paleo House, for breakfast at Emma and Tim's instigation. I follow the Paleo regime, with some modifications, and I'm touched that the children are prepared to pander to what I'm sure they consider to be 'Mum's weird dietary habits.' Fortunately the food is delicious and we all enjoy our meals.

I'm amazed at how well all the children have coped with the news. I must have done a good job at convincing them I'm going to be fine—or maybe I've bred a tribe of stoics.

In the early afternoon when Emma and Tim go home, they leave a big aching hole and all the light has gone out of the day. It takes me back to my childhood, when my grandmother, whom I loved dearly, would come to stay with our family for a few days. After we waved her off, I would spend the day wandering aimlessly around in the vast, lonely silence she had left behind.

The next day is my first day back at work after my diagnosis. Telling my co-workers is tough. I send out a brief email outlining the facts, so I don't have to tell the same story multiple times. Then I go to lunch so I'm not around when they read it. When I return, I get lots of sympathetic comments and hugs, bringing more tears to my eyes.

I don't think there would be anyone who'd disagree that breaking the news about your cancer diagnosis isn't harrowing, particularly as you're still in shock yourself. Over time, I find that telling others about my diagnosis helps me to come to terms with it and accept that it's real.

Rochelle was 32 when diagnosed. Her friends and family were shocked at her diagnosis, due to her age and fitness as a triathlete. When she first broke the news, she referred to a 'lump in my breast that is cancerous'. She knew it had finally hit home when she was able to say, 'I have breast cancer.'

There can be amusing moments too. Yvonne's sons were 13 and 11 when she was diagnosed. 'I sat them down and told them about my diagnosis, and that I had to go into hospital but that I would be okay. I was very careful about what I said, putting a positive spin on it, so they wouldn't be too upset. When I'd finished, I asked them if they had any questions.'

'Yes,' they said, 'can we go and skate now?'

The resilience of children!

I think it would be very difficult to break the news of cancer to young children—you don't want them to be too upset or their lives to be too disrupted, and it's tricky to achieve that fine balance between relaying the facts and giving them comfort and reassurance. No matter what you say, children pick up very easily on anxiety and fear, and I'm very thankful I don't have the extra responsibility of young children to cope with.

*

The next two weeks until we leave for our holiday are difficult. There's lots of conversation, both at work and with family and friends, about my diagnosis and what's in store for me, but it still hasn't hit home. One of the reasons is that unlike many illnesses, breast cancer is usually asymptomatic – until you start treatment.

I still look and feel as fit and healthy as ever, and I continue my usual activities including going to the gym. It's hard to imagine there's a foreign, malignant mass inside me and I feel that somehow other people can see it—that I'll be stopped at Customs in the US by an official saying, 'I'm sorry Madam, but you can't come into the country with that lump. You'll have to get rid of it first.'

I'm drowning in information—besides the books I've been given from the Cancer Council, I have also signed up as a member of Breast Cancer Network of Australia, and they send me more information: a Pilates CD and a journal called My Journey in which to record my experiences. I read as much of the information as I can take in because I like to be informed about what's going on in my body and what my treatment choices are. I've always been proactive when it comes to my health.

Which has got me wondering why I got breast cancer—not as

in weeping and gnashing of teeth, and wailing to the heavens 'Why me?'

But more like a miffed 'I've been the epitome of health – I'm not overweight, I eat well, exercise regularly, drink moderately and don't smoke. I can't remember the last time I had a cold or the flu. I'm just a wee bit annoyed about this, Universe. And to add insult to injury, I've never taken my good health for granted. There's been many a time when I've encountered others with severe health issues and given thanks for my good health. I've even been a regular blood donor so that others can benefit from my wellbeing. And this is how you repay me! It's enough to make me want to lie around on the couch all day stuffing myself with fried chicken and ice-cream sundaes!'

But there's been one part of my wholesome clean-living life that hasn't been ideal. Stress. Stress in itself is not inherently bad if it's related to something you enjoy—it motivates and challenges you, and makes you productive. When it's related to something you don't enjoy, it can become harmful.

I'm no longer getting any satisfaction from my work as a probation and parole officer, and my efforts to cope with the stress haven't always been successful. How stress affects us is such an individual thing that it's almost impossible to establish a causal link between it and any disease. Even proving it's a contributing factor is difficult. But I figure that because stress affects our immune system, which in turn affects how our body reacts to abnormal cell growth, it has to play some part.

I come to the conclusion that although stress may well have played a part in my getting breast cancer, it's not the whole story and there's probably nothing I could have done to prevent it. It's our human need to control our lives that makes us think otherwise. A diagnosis of breast cancer brings home to us that there are many aspects of our lives that are out of our control.

And I'm wondering if my gratitude for my good health was like a red flag to those contrary Gods of Health. Perhaps they misinterpreted it as complacency and decided to teach me a lesson. 'You think you're healthy? Cop this and see how you feel!'

I've learned my lesson; you can stop now!

Kath, who like me led a healthy lifestyle, tells a story of attending a nursing conference. A whole segment was devoted to the study of the breast, with the statistics quoted that 1 in 14 women were diagnosed with breast cancer. (That was 21 years ago; the incidence is now 1 in 8).

'I remember looking around at everyone else there and thinking smugly, "Well, it won't be me."'

A year later, she was diagnosed with breast cancer. Those Gods of Health have one helluva sense of humour.

The First Cut Is
Not The Deepest

We're finally on the plane to Los Angeles, to be followed by a short flight to San Diego. Some people have said, 'Why don't you postpone your trip until after your treatment is finished? Then you'll be able to enjoy it more.'

But I'm glad I don't take their advice. Apart from the fact that we would miss the conference on internet marketing (which will help both Aaron's business and my writing) if we postponed the trip, I want more than ever to have a holiday and take a breather from the events of the last three weeks.

It's the right decision. We have a fantastic time—with new places to see and new experiences to enjoy every day, I forget a lot of the time that I even have breast cancer. When I do remember, I quickly put it to the back of my mind. 'I'll deal with it when I get back,' I tell myself. I'm a master of procrastination and this time it stands me in good stead.

The day we return home from our trip, tired and jet-lagged, we receive some news that changes my life. Before we left, I submitted a claim to my insurance company to be paid a lump sum in accordance with my critical illness insurance policy. The company phones to tell us my claim has been accepted and the full amount has already been deposited into our bank account. With whoops of joy, we go to check. Sure enough it's there.

This six-figure sum means I can resign from my job and use it as income for the next three years, so I can become a full-time author—with money left over for other uses. I feel as if I've won the lottery.

I've often heard people say that getting cancer, or some other serious illness, was the best thing that happened to them because it was a wake-up call that forced them to take stock of their lives and change it for the better. And that further, if they had their time over, they would still choose their illness. I used to think that was crazy—if you had a choice, wouldn't you choose to be well? And if you had to have a wake-up call, have it by some other means?

But now I know what they mean. I've been a part-time author for many years, and it's been my dream to quit my job to write full time. But I haven't had the guts to do it because we've needed my income, although to be perfectly truthful, it's also been due to a fear of failure – that I wouldn't be able to make it work.

Now this opportunity has been given to me, courtesy of breast cancer. Gift-wrapped in pink, with a large pink bow and presented to me with a tag saying, 'To Robin, Enclosed please find three years to do with whatever you want'. Thank you, Gods of Health. I take it all back.

What a weight has been lifted off my shoulders—a weight I didn't even realise was there because I was so used to it. And when three years is up? Who knows? Anything could happen during that time. That's as far ahead as I want to think at the moment.

*

A week later, I have an appointment at the hospital with my surgeon, whom I'll meet for the first time. Aaron comes with me.

We're called into the consulting room and I look around

while we're waiting for him to appear. American humourist Erma Bombeck, who also had breast cancer, was quoted as saying, 'Never go to a doctor whose office plants have died'.

Fortunately there are no plants in the room, which either means he never had any, or he had some and they died—and he's quickly removed the evidence so none of his patients are any the wiser.

While I'm hoping that the first is the correct reason, the surgeon arrives, introducing himself as Scott. He's young and fresh-faced, with blue eyes and a gentle and compassionate manner. And warm hands. I know this because I didn't flinch as he examined my breast. (Hand temperature should be one of the criteria for entrance into medical school). In fact, if I were 30 years younger, I'd probably have a crush on him. I wonder if he's married—thinking of my 28-year-old-unattached daughter. Maybe he could be my son-in-law. But how many men could admit to having felt their mother-in-law's breast? Forget that idea.

Scott informs me that he is a part of my breast cancer team, consisting of all the medical staff involved in my treatment, from the breast care nurse to the oncologist. They have meetings every Friday, discuss my case and make recommendations for treatment tailored to my particular diagnosis and circumstances.

I'm impressed. I like the idea of having a team behind me— like a sports team, someone to barrack for me and get me over the finish line. And my inner egotist likes the idea of being the topic of discussion, even if I can't be present to enjoy it.

'You have a choice of treatment,' Scott says. Breast conserving surgery—removal of the lump and one lymph gland for testing—or a mastectomy. Breast conserving surgery is usually recommended for early stage breast cancer and is the one recommended by my team. (I'm flattered—they've discussed me already!) The advantage of a mastectomy is that you usually don't need radiation therapy afterwards, or have to worry about the cancer recurring in that breast.

For me, losing a breast is too high a price to pay for those advantages. I'm happy to do radiation therapy, and Scott assures me that I'll be regularly monitored after treatment so that if there's any recurrence, it will be picked up early. I'm a minimal interventionist when it comes to medical issues.

I look at Aaron. I know what he's thinking. 'I don't need to think about it,' I say. 'I'll take the breast conservation surgery.'

Then we go home to wait for the advice of my surgery date. I dive in straight away into my new career, structuring my time so that I'm writing during the day, and doing administration and marketing activities at night. A week later, I receive a letter informing me of the date in three weeks for my lumpectomy, or 'procedure' in medicalspeak.

Procedure is such a satisfyingly vague term. It could mean anything from an ingrown toenail to an amputation. Tell people you're going into hospital for a procedure and they look uncertain and a little alarmed. Not game to ask what it is (because surely if you'd wanted them to know, you'd have told them) but not sure whether to be happy for you, or to commiserate with you.

As well as removing the lump, the surgeon will also remove my first lymph node (called a sentinel node biopsy) to test for cancer as this is the first place it will go to if it has spread. On the day before my lumpectomy, I attend an X-ray clinic to have some radioactive blue dye injected into my breast, which will travel to the lymph node to help the surgeon identify and remove it.

My breast is now a fetching bright blue. I then have to lie very still under the X-ray machine while it takes 3D photos. It's a large tunnel-like machine that revolves around me. I wonder if you have to wear those 3D goggles you get at the movies to look at the photos. It feels very space-agey, and I have a vision of the large plates suddenly breaking loose and clamping down on top of me, flattening me into a pancake.

The next morning, Aaron drives me to the hospital and stays with me until I get called into the treatment room for the insertion of the hookwire. I give him an extra long kiss and watch him as he walks back down the hallway. That could be our last kiss if something goes wrong on the operating table. This might sound melodramatic for a simple, hour-long operation, but I've never had any major illnesses or been in hospital since the birth of my youngest child 24 years ago. In addition, I have a fear of going under general anaesthetic and not coming out the other end, that fear of loss of control again.

Having the hookwire inserted into my breast soon takes my mind off my imminent death. It's as unpleasant as it sounds as the local anaesthetic doesn't completely mask the pain. The hookwire is a marker for the surgeon to find the lump. By now it's occurred to me that contrary to my supposition, the lump is not discernible to the naked eye from the rest of the breast tissue. For the surgeons, it must be like going into a dark tunnel without a light and trying to find a pebble on the floor. Then I'm taken into the surgical waiting room inhabited by a handful of other patients also dressed in the fetching puke-green hospital gowns, support stockings and orange socks.

And there I wait. And wait. I try to keep my mind occupied to deflect my anxiety. I read trashy magazines and watch infomercials on the TV, the intellectual equivalent of junk food, until my brain is bloated. I wonder what my fellow patients are in for. The old man next to me has fallen asleep and is snoring, so he's obviously not too concerned. Perhaps an ingrown toenail?

Scott pops in to check that I'm okay. 'Shouldn't be long,' he says. Which in medicalspeak means: 'As soon as we've dealt with all the emergencies, had afternoon tea and found the anaesthetist'.

My stomach is protesting loudly. As per the instructions, I haven't eaten or drunk anything all day; and I start to hallucinate strong, rich coffee and dark, melt-in-your-mouth sea salt chocolate.

After four and a half hours of waiting, I'm called into the pre-op room where I meet my anaesthetist Frank, a friendly grey-

haired man. He asks me my name, date of birth and what I'm
having done, for what seems like the thousandth time that day. I
assume it's to make sure they're doing the right thing to the
right person.

I remember my mother (whose quirky sense of humour I've
inherited) telling me that when she was in hospital to have her
varicose veins stripped, the anaesthetist asked her the usual
questions and she said, 'It's the left leg being amputated, isn't
it?' Which caused the anaesthetist to look at her sharply and
check his notes ——just in case.

'It would serve you right,' I told my mother, 'if he went ahead
and cut off your left leg, just to teach you a lesson.'

When Aaron recently underwent day surgery and the anaesthetist asked him what he was in for, he said, 'A new head. My
missus doesn't like this one, says it's getting a bit old and bat-
tered.'

The anaesthetist roared with laughter. 'You've made my day!'
he said and walked off chuckling and muttering, 'A new head!'

I guess when you have a job where everyone you meet is putting their life in your hands, any light relief is welcome.

Frank then regales me with all sorts of family anecdotes,
probably to take my mind off the fact that he's making several
painful attempts to insert a canula into my forearm—a common
problem, apparently, as the veins shrink due to dehydration. We
both give a sigh of relief when he finally succeeds. I find that
slow, deep breathing helps to calm me, especially after he goes
away and leaves me alone on the bed contemplating my fate.

I reflect that it's so trusting of the doctors to leave me alone
in a room full of medical apparatus. What if my anxiety causes
me to have a brain snap; and I spring off my bed, pull out my
canula and rifle through all the drawers, arming myself with
syringes and drugs and bandages and running amok through
the hospital? Or (which is more likely for me) what if I just
quietly slip off my bed and sneak into the nearest restroom and
hide? Do I have an overactive imagination or do other people

entertain these sorts of fantasies as well?

When I'm finally wheeled into the operation room, it's even more scary. I feel very vulnerable as I stare up at the huge lights beaming down on me like mini flying saucers, while a bunch of gowned and masked figures mill around me. It's like a scene from a TV medical drama and I imagine myself saying in a small voice, 'I will be all right, won't I doctor?'

And the doctor exchanging meaningful glances with his medical team (because everyone except the patient knows that this is SERIOUS) before patting my hand and saying, 'Everything will be just fine.'

Then someone is shaking me and saying, 'Wake up, Robin.'

It's all over and I'm still alive.

*

That night Aaron visits me and brings me roses. Apart from a little soreness, I feel fine. And euphoric that it's over. I'm in a public ward; and after he goes, I spend the night checking out the nurses and my fellow patients (in a surreptitious manner, of course—I'm a writer, it's part of the job description) and eavesdropping on their conversations. Not much point in trying to sleep—it's like being in bed in the middle of peak hour traffic.

It becomes obvious that my procedure was minor compared to the afflictions of my fellow wardmates. One woman moans all night with pain; the man beside me, who fell off a roof and broke his ribs, discovered during a routine CT scan of his brain that he has a brain tumour; and the man on the other side of me has serious kidney problems.

Thank God I only have breast cancer.

My Cancer Cells Have The Travel Bug

On my discharge the next morning from hospital, I'm given an appointment for ten days time to see Scott and get the results from the lumpectomy and lymph node removal.

Over the next few days, I take it easy even though my first impulse is to plunge back into my normal routine as I feel well, apart from a little soreness in the breast. But I've been warned about being too complacent. I'm conscientious about doing the arm and shoulder exercises given to me by the hospital physiotherapist to get movement back and to minimise the risk of lymphedema.

A premonition hovers in the back of my mind all week. I'm confident that the lymph node will be clear, but I have an intuition that the other results won't be straightforward—that there will be something not right about them. But I don't verbalise my fears as I know people will only say, 'Don't worry, I'm sure you'll be fine'. They say those things to try and make you feel better, but of course they don't know at all.

As Aaron and I sit in the surgical outpatients waiting area of the hospital, I look around. All the other patients look the part—

they're on crutches or in wheelchairs, coughing, wheezing and rasping or just looking generally unhealthy. Compared to them, I'm a picture of health and vitality, as if I've just stepped off the cover of *Good Health* magazine. I feel like an imposter. They're probably looking at me wondering what's wrong with me.

It's a feeling I have many times over the course of my treatment, and it's a bit of a trap. Because I look and feel so well, I can kid myself that this cancer is just a small blip on my health radar and that I'll be over it in no time. Which doesn't allow for the emotional aspects—the tears, fears and sadness that can appear out of the blue.

We're called into Scott's consulting room, and I find out that my intuition is correct. 'The lymph node was clear,' he says. 'But unfortunately we found DCIS cells in the lump. Although the margins were clear, we're concerned that some of those cells may have travelled further into the breast. So we'd like to take some more tissue out for testing, just to make sure.'

I'm trying to take it all in. What are DCIS cells? He's talking as if I should know what they are. They must be serious if he's talking in initials. Initials mean that the word is long and complicated, which translated means 'not good'.

'I'm pretty sure the results will be good,' Scott is saying. 'But the only way we can be certain is to do another procedure.' I'll be notified of a date; he thinks it will be in about three weeks.

Aaron and I are sombre on the way home. 'I was expecting something like this,' I say and tell him about my premonition.

The fact that I have to undergo another procedure has taken the gloss off the good news that the cancer hasn't spread to the lymph glands. But we try to put a good spin on it, telling ourselves that I'm lucky the doctors are so thorough—after all, don't I also want to be reassured that those pesky DCIS cells haven't packed their microscopic suitcases and gone on a tour through the rest of my breast?

When I get home, I consult the ever-reliable Dr Google and discover that DCIS stands for ductal carcinoma in situ and they are the abnormal, pre-cancerous cells, which may or may not end up as fully fledged cancer cells. But when you already have cancer, you don't want any baby cancer cells lurking around.

So begins more waiting, conveying the news to family and friends and trying to remain positive for their sake as much as mine. I attend a follow-up appointment with the physiotherapist, and the good news is I have regained full use of my arm and shoulder (which I knew already) so I don't have to do the exercises any more. I also have the go-ahead to resume my body balance and yoga classes. I'm as happy as a kid with a good report card—A+ for health!

The second procedure is day surgery only, though still under general anaesthetic, and there's no dye or hookwire involved. All goes according to plan. I thought I would be less anxious about the operation this time as at least I now know what's involved, but not so. My usual deep breathing techniques stand me in good stead; it's impossible to feel anxious when you're deep breathing as it slows your heart rate down. At home that night, I rummage around in the kitchen like a scavenging wolf, appeasing my day-long fast.

I've booked to attend a workshop, *Between the Sheets*, on erotic writing at a local library the following day, which I organised before I knew my operation date. Not that I'm planning a career as a writer of erotica, but I'm hoping that it will equip me with the tools (sorry, skills) to write evocative and original love scenes, something I've always found challenging. As I'm feeling fine, I decide to still go. Aaron has offered to take me, as I'm not allowed to drive for the next 24 hours.

All the attendees at the workshop are women, which is not surprising. There must be male erotica writers but they're probably still in the closet, scribbling away in the dark. It's very hands-on (I mean, practical) with plenty of writing exercises. These consume my full powers of concentration—it would be hard to pick a less sexy time for a woman than when she has just had a piece gouged out of her breast, which now resembles a warped, deflated, bright blue party balloon. One of the exercises is to write an erotic scene in which one of the characters has a bodily imperfection. I consider writing about someone with a mangled breast but decide against it. It's too raw at the moment.

The workshop is very enlightening and I'm glad I made the effort to attend. Later that day, I'm amused to learn there was an earth tremor in the area, big enough to rattle doors and windows, and shake furniture. None of us in the class had any idea—we were outside on the lawn doing a group writing exercise. So the earth moved and none of us felt it. A reflection of our erotic writing skills, perhaps?

*

I turn 60 the day before my appointment to get my test results. Apart from phone calls and messages, it's just a normal day. I do some writing in the local library, which has become my away-from-home office and go to the gym in the afternoon. Before my diagnosis, I had vague hopes of a party or a night out in an upmarket restaurant, but now celebrations seem unimportant.

Aaron and I go out for dinner the following Saturday night, and I discover that my eldest daughter Emma has booked and paid for us – her brother Tim, Aaron and me – to spend a weekend in a five-star resort in Byron Bay, a popular coastal town about three hours drive away, as a birthday present. I'm very moved and so happy that I have something to look forward to. It beats a party or a dinner any day.

Although Scott has said he's confident the test results will be clear, my stomach has been churning all day. Whether it's just anxiety or my intuition at work, I don't know. But there's good reason for it, as I find out.

As Scott is away, we see another doctor—a young woman who breaks the news gently. 'The tissue was clear but the margins weren't. We could do another procedure but our recommendation is for you to have a mastectomy.'

As the news sinks in, tears spring to my eyes. This is the worst possible news. Not for one moment have I thought that this would be a possibility. I clutch at the only straw I can see.

'But there's an option to have another procedure?'

'Yes, but we can't guarantee the appearance of your breast after a third procedure.'

The doctor explains that my team has recommended a mastectomy purely on cosmetic grounds. If I were to have more tissue taken out and the results were clear, my prognosis would be no worse than if I'd had a mastectomy.

'But as I said before, after another procedure, the appearance of your breast may be severely compromised.'

I look at Aaron. I know he's thinking exactly the same as me. 'The way I look at it, half a boob is better than none at all,' I proclaim with attempted bravado.

'Although a mastectomy is our recommendation, the decision is yours,' the doctor says, 'and we'll respect it, whatever it is. However, I must warn you that if you choose to have another procedure, and the test results are not clear, we won't do another one. A mastectomy will be your only option.'

She makes another appointment for next week, by which time I need to have made my decision.

Mastectomy Or Not

Over the next week, I feel as if my emotions are going through an endless washing machine cycle. Fast, slow, rinse, spin and repeat. I only have seven days to make a decision that will affect the rest of my life.

My gut reaction as soon as the doctor told us the options was to choose the further procedure. Not only is it in line with my minimalist intervention philosophy but if there's a chance to save my breast, I want to take it. My concern is more with my body's health than its appearance. My days of topless sunbaking are well and truly over; I can live with the knowledge that I'll never win a wet t-shirt competition and Aaron is the only person likely to see my breast (apart from the doctors), and he doesn't care what it looks like as long as I'm alive. If the test results come back as positive next time, I'll be willing to go ahead with a mastectomy, knowing that I've done everything I can to avoid it.

Even so, my mind still runs round in circles, agonising over whether it's the right decision. But I keep coming back to the same scenario: if I decide to have a mastectomy and the test results come back clear, I'd feel upset and cheated that I'd lost my breast when it wasn't necessary.

I ask my father, who retired as a general practitioner 25 years ago, for his opinion. 'I'd advise you to have the mastectomy,' he says. But he can't give a logical reason, other than it's the cancer team's recommendation.

The other males in my life don't venture an opinion, undoubtedly feeling that it's totally out of their league—like me giving an opinion on whether they should have a testicle removed. Except Aaron, of course, who is of the same frame of mind as me. The women, on the other hand, are more than happy to give me the benefit of their mostly unsolicited advice. Surprisingly, most say they'd opt for the mastectomy.

'What use are my boobs now?' says one middle-aged, well-endowed relative. 'They just get in the way. If it were me I'd say, "Take them both off."'

'What have you got against a mastectomy anyway?' asks another, in the same tone of voice as you might discuss my aversion to brussels sprouts or rap music. I burn with indignation. 'You go and have one if you think it's so easy,' I want to shout at her.

One thing I do have against a mastectomy is that I'm very attached to my breasts. They've been with me through thick and thin, ever since I started growing them at 12 and asked my mother to take me bra shopping. I'd just started my first year at boarding school and was mortified to find that I was the only girl in my dormitory not wearing a bra—and some of them were flatter than me.

My mother said the worst thing you could say to an almost teenager. 'But you've got nothing to put in a bra!' And then, 'I didn't wear one till I was 17!'

I looked at her with disbelief. Either she was an extremely late developer (which I doubted) or she'd been going around for years with her breasts jiggling freely within her prim, neck-to-knee school uniform, before they were finally restrained behind bras. I hastily expunged this disturbing image from my mind.

Mum eventually gave in to my pleading and took me bra shopping, insisting that I be properly fitted by an expert. I wanted to shrivel into a ball of embarrassment as the motherly bra-fitting lady in the department store trotted in and out of the change room with various bras, pummelling and pushing me into them, adjusting the straps and standing back to survey me. Wasn't there a way she could fit me with the proper size without me having to expose my naked breasts? Couldn't she just poke the bras through the curtain with her eyes closed, let me put my own bra on and then come in when I shouted 'Ready'?

From that point on, I insisted on buying my own bras. Over the next few years, my breasts served the usual functions of being ogled and gawped at, creating a bit of cleavage when out to impress and being exposed to the elements on the odd occasion I was brave enough to go topless sunbathing.

But they really came into their own after I married and had children. They fed my three children for the first twelve or so months of their lives; and in their first three months, they grew as fat as toads exclusively on my breastmilk. I realise that not all mothers feel that way about breastfeeding –– some have problems and others don't enjoy it. I would never judge another mother for not breastfeeding, whatever the reason, but I took to it like a cow to the milking machine.

Back in the 1980s, when I had my children, demand feeding had hit its straps. The philosophy was to feed babies when they were hungry, however often that was, but our parents were of the generation that believed in putting babies on a four-hourly feeding schedule. If they woke up after three hours crying, you were supposed to let them cry for another hour before you fed them.

Unfortunately, a lot of babies hadn't read the manual about four-hourly feeding—mine certainly hadn't. As an adult, I don't go four hours without eating. It was a lot easier and less stressful just to feed the babies when they cried—and nine times out of ten it was because they were hungry. But both my mother and my mother-in-law were disapproving. 'Are you feeding her again? You're exhausting yourself! Why don't you put her on the bottle?'

What was exhausting about it? You're forced to sit down when you breastfeed, you get to see a lot of TV; and if you've got it set up properly, you can read a book and drink a glass of wine (only if it's after 5pm of course) at the same time. With children numbers two and three, breastfeeding was a good time for the other child/children to sit beside me on the couch and have a book read to them. The best part of all is the oxytocin, the hormone that's released when you're breastfeeding. It relaxes you and gives you a wonderful sense of calm and peace. Someone should find a way of bottling and selling it—much better for you than alcohol or drugs.

As for putting my children on the bottle, they wouldn't have a bar of it. I tried briefly with all of them, hoping that I could express some milk into a bottle, hire a babysitter and have the occasional night out; but when I put the teat in their mouths, they curled up their little lips in distaste, like a wine connoisseur who'd just been offered a cleanskin from the bargain bin and with a cry that clearly said, 'What? You can't be serious, surely?'

When I had my third child, I intended to breastfeed him for as long as he wanted as I knew he was my last. But he had other ideas. At ten months, he woke up one morning and refused to feed. No amount of persuasion could change his mind—I even considered coating my nipple in chocolate. He'd obviously decided that life sucked being dependent on the tit, and it was time to man up and swig out of a cup, which he promptly did. Giving up breastfeeding suddenly is not a good idea as it can lead to mastitis, but as I had no choice, it was off to the doctor to get some pills to dry up my milk.

So after their finest hours, my breasts went the way of every woman's as she gets older—southwards. But not too much. One advantage of being on the small side is that when your boobs start to droop, it's not as noticeable. Where would we be without push-up bras!

I survey my breasts in the mirror. I've taken them for granted for all these years, but now I see them in a new light and they look pretty damned good. I don't even add the proviso 'for their age', as I've seen breasts on 20-year-olds that were less perky than mine.

Even the breast that's in danger of being lopped off is not too bad. It's still blue from the dye injection, a bit puckered and asymmetrical, with a semi-circular scar at the base as if it's smiling, but it's still a breast. Like something Picasso would paint.

As I'm pondering the issue, I realise there's one very important question I forgot to ask the doctor—if I go ahead with another procedure, what are the chances of the test results being positive? If the odds were high, I would rethink my decision, but I wonder whether the doctor is able or prepared to make an educated guess. However, none of them have a crystal ball, and in the end that's all it would be—a guess.

To help me make the decision, I have booked a phone consultation with a nurse counsellor, one of the many services offered by the Cancer Council in my state. Trudy is very careful not to express an opinion herself. Nevertheless, she helps me to not only confirm that having another procedure rather than a mastectomy is the right course of action for me, but also to have confidence in my decision. As much as I try not to be swayed by others' opinions, it still takes courage to go against them as well as medical advice, particularly when I'm feeling so vulnerable. I could live with others not agreeing with my decision, but I knew I couldn't live with not being true to my own wishes.

Uncertainty Is
A Certainty

It turns out that Scott is very accepting of my decision and has no qualms about carrying out another procedure. 'We'll do the best we can to conserve as much of the breast as possible,' he says in his calm, laid-back manner, which goes a long way towards reassuring me. When asked about the odds of the next test result being positive, he says, 'I think the results will be fine.'

He also answers the list of questions I've brought in with me, including the Big Curly Question—is this going to kill me, if not now then further down the track? 'You're not going to die from this,' he assures me. 'We're looking at a cure here.'

It's very refreshing and heartening to have a doctor who's so positive, as many are either non-committal or give you the worst-case scenario—I guess in order not to raise your hopes. However, as far as the outcome of the next procedure goes, I'm trying not to have any expectations despite Scott's positive predictions. After all, he was wrong last time. One thing I've learnt is that expectations can cause a lot of distress if they don't come to fruition. I need to protect myself in the event of a bad outcome.

While I'm waiting to be advised of my hospital date for the procedure, I have my weekend away to Byron Bay with the family. On the way, we call in to see a friend at Murwillumbah. Stuart, in his early fifties, has been diagnosed with bone marrow cancer.

'I cried for two days when I first found out,' he says. He was originally given a prognosis of five to seven years, but because he's so fit and it's been diagnosed early, his doctor thinks it's more likely to be fifteen.

"I'll take the fifteen,' he grins. As cancer patients we have an instant bond, but not for the first time I'm grateful for having breast cancer, as opposed to any other form of cancer. I'm also mindful of the fact that just because I've been told I'll be cured and Stuart's been given 15 years means nothing in the long run. Who knows how long any of us have on this earth? It's unwise to become too complacent.

Our weekend at Byron Bay is wonderful and restorative for body and soul at a time when it's just what I need—lots of eating, drinking, swimming, walking and laughing. And lots of jokes about playing the 'cancer card,' though in reality I would never do that to get sympathy or special treatment (except to get out of washing the dishes).

When we return from Byron Bay, I'm given the date for my procedure in two weeks. I also have an MRI scheduled for next week—another routine test to see if any more reprobate cancer cells are hiding in my breast, particularly any DCIS cells. I've never had an MRI and am warned I may find it traumatic if I am claustrophobic, which I am. The receptionist advises me to take a sedative beforehand, but I decide not to as I'll be incapable of driving home afterwards. I'll just close my eyes and deep breathe my way through it.

As it turns out, claustrophobia isn't an issue as I'm lying on the stretcher on my stomach with my face firmly embedded in a padded hole, similar to a massage table, so I can't see a thing anyway. My breasts are poking through two holes in the stretcher, and a bizarre image pops into my mind of what this must look like from below, if anyone happened to be lurking underneath. I've brought along a CD of meditation music to be played through my headphones, but the calming effect is negated by the constant barrage of noises reverberating in my head, ranging from a baritone jackhammer to a high-pitched wail, as the machine does its job. They sound like a cross between a tone-deaf orchestra tuning up and a torture chamber for the hearing-impaired. When the technicians finally wheel me out of the tunnel, I have an urge to sit up and yell, 'Okay, I confess! I killed him!'

*

On the morning of the operation, a Friday, I wake up depressed. We've had relatives staying for the past few days; and with all the accompanying socialising, I haven't had time to think about it. But now they've all left and reality has kicked in. Aaron goes to work and I pull the sheets back over me, and hide under them until 8.30, when I make myself get up and do some chores.

Aaron comes to pick me up and I'm at the hospital at the appointed time of 12.30 pm. But due to some emergency surgeries, I've been demoted to last on the list, although they don't tell me that until they whisk me into the pre-operating theatre at 4.45 pm—by which time I've already come to that conclusion. I'm hoping they're not going to do a rushed job and forget to do something vital, like sewing me up again, so they can get away for the weekend.

The anaesthetist, a younger one this time, again has trouble putting in the canula; but his boss gets one in on the third attempt, leaving the other two failures still in my hand. Then they both disappear, leaving me resembling some avant-garde work of art lying there with three needles sticking out of my hand. Another Picasso perhaps? Or something more contemporary: Woman With Needles – An Exposition of Drug Abuse. I'm still as nervous as I was the first time, so I practise my deep breath-ing until I'm wheeled into the operating room.

Scott comes over and squeezes my hand. 'How are you?' he asks.

'Fine,' I say brightly, 'I'm an old hand now; I can do this with my eyes closed.'

I'm disappointed that he doesn't even smile at my joke, but maybe he's heard it countless times before. For some reason I feel as if I have a responsibility to reassure him that I'm okay, I can get through this and cracking jokes is part of that. It's a reversal of roles—instead of him telling me I'll be okay, I'm reassuring him. I don't want him worrying needlessly about me, wondering if I'm going to go gaga with the stress of it all.

I'm not the only one who feels the need to be funny in the operating room. The day before her mastectomy, Kay treated herself to a morning at the hairdresser's. She was also having a breast reconstruction at the same time and knew that after ten hours on the operating table, she wasn't going to be looking her best. If nothing else, she decided at least she'd have great hair.

When she got to the pre-operating room on the day, Kay told the anaesthetist she was nervous; so he gave her a pill, telling her it was a relaxant. To this day she doesn't know what it was, but the effect was similar to a couple of strong cocktails. As she was wheeled into the operating room, everyone in the medical fraternity was there: oncologist, surgeon, plastic surgeon, two anaesthetists and all their assistants, and a sprinkling of nurs-es—maybe even the cleaner and the tea lady as well. They were all standing together looking at a large computer screen, no doubt checking the last minute important details—like which breast they were going to take off.

'Hi everyone!" Kay called out, waving merrily. 'I just wanted to let you know I've had my hair done for the occasion.' They all turned around, smiled perfunctorily and turned back to the screen.

Now everyone knows that when a woman tells you she's had

her hair done, you don't just smile and turn away. The correct response is, 'You look fantastic—it really suits you.' At the bare minimum.

But Kay, to her credit, didn't get upset. Which probably had a lot to do with the 'relaxant'. She just ramped it up a bit.

'I'm not kidding,' she called out, even louder. 'I really have had my hair done for this occasion.'

'That's the last thing I remembered,' she told me later. 'I think they must have knocked me out pretty quickly.'

*

The procedure goes according to plan and I go home that night. My appointment with the surgeon to get the test results is the next Thursday, six days away. There's a lump of dread in the pit of my stomach—I'm thinking that the results will not be clear. My hunches have all been right up to this point, but it could just be that I'm protecting myself against disappointment and preparing for the worst.

I've been reading a book by Dr Susan Jeffers called *Embracing Uncertainty*. It's an excellent book that I can highly recommend to anyone, especially those with cancer, as often our journey seems to be one uncertainty after another. Humans have a basic need for security and safety and we like to feel that we're in control, but uncertainty is a fact of life and there are many things that are outside our sphere of control. In fact, Dr Jeffers argues that we have no control over our future at all and that instead of fearing and worrying about uncertainty, we need to welcome and embrace it, as only then can we achieve true peace of mind.

She also discusses expectations and how they can derail us and set us up for disappointment and misery. In one exercise, she challenges us to change the words 'I hope' to 'I wonder', thereby leaving us open to whatever the outcome may be. At first it's not easy to do with any sense of conviction, but I give it a go. Instead of saying to myself, 'I hope the test results are clear,' I say, 'I wonder if the test results will be clear.'

But it's negated by the fact that I'm telling myself they won't be.

I Can See Clearly Now

Once more, Aaron and I are sitting in the surgical outpatients waiting area. It's been a long wait and I've read the same page of the gossip magazine three times. Finally, the breast care nurse comes hurrying out and beckons us in.

'Good news,' she tells us before we even reach the consulting room. 'The test results were clear.'

'Yes!' Aaron says, doing a fist pump. 'I knew they would be!' And he did. He's been telling me all week they'd be clear. I'm stunned; I can't take it in.

Scott confirms the results and has a look at his handiwork. He's done a magnificent job—the scar is not noticeably larger than before and there's still plenty of breast left, enough to fill a bra cup without having to resort to tissue stuffing. Clearly he was underestimating his skills if he thought he would leave me with a mangled breast.

'Thank you so much,' I tell him. 'I'm so glad I made the decision not to have a mastectomy.' We say goodbye to him for another six months until my next check-up. I'm now in the hands of the radiotherapy team.

It takes the rest of the day for the good news to sink in, and telling family and friends helps the process. I've learnt that my intuition is not infallible, and I'm glad it was wrong on this occasion. I'm walking on air and brimming with clarity and energy. I review the five-year plan I've made for my career as an author, crystallise my goals and give them time frames. The idea for this book *Making The Breast Of It* has been germinating over the last couple of weeks, and now I sit down and make a rough outline.

I also join the online community of the Breast Cancer Network of Australia, hoping to connect with women willing to share their experiences with me for the book. So many women, so many stories, each one unique. I feel an affinity with all of them, that if we met on the street, we would have an immediate connection. But I guess it's the same for any group of people who have undergone a harrowing experience together, especially one that touches on our mortality.

It reminds us of our humanity, that we all experience the same hopes and fears, and in a group such as this, you focus on what you have in common and accept what you don't. Sounds like a pretty good recipe for world peace.

Radiating Joy

The next thing on the agenda is an appointment with the radiation oncology team. The oncologist outlines how radiation therapy (also called radiotherapy) works. In a nutshell, it's a special kind of high-energy beam, invisible to the naked eye, that damages the DNA of the cancer cells so they are unable to reproduce. He also recommends four weeks of treatment instead of the six weeks I was originally advised.

'Recent studies have shown that four weeks is just as effective as six weeks,' he says. I'm not about to argue with that. He also tells me I have the choice of undertaking chemotherapy as well if I want to. However it makes my prognosis only marginally better and his opinion is that I don't need it. I'm happy to go along with that too; I can't see the point of undergoing the trauma of it for such a miniscule benefit. To my way of thinking, it's like trying to kill an ant with a machine gun. Leave the big guns for a time when I might need them—hopefully never.

Later in the week, I have an appointment with the medical imaging team at the hospital to have a CT scan and tattoos. These help the radiation therapists to pinpoint the exact area that needs to be treated, as the beams must be directed at the same spot each time to be effective. The tattoos are rather painful and the reason why I will never get real ones—I'm a wimp when it comes to pain. Don't ask me how I managed to give birth to three children.

At the end of the procedure, I have a cross on both sides of my breast for a religious flavour and a dot at each end of my scar, one on my chest and one at the top of my ribs, like some bizarre game of join the dots. To add insult to injury, they also take my photo, which I'm not happy about as I suffer from Photo Drug Face Syndrome. As soon as an official photo is imminent, my eyes glaze over, my mouth purses itself into a surly line; and I look as if I'm recovering from a torrid night of partying with illicit substances—an especially good look for a passport photo.

Then yet another appointment, this time for a bone density scan. I fully understand women who refer to their breast cancer treatment as their new full-time occupation. There are always appointments, consultations, piles of material to read, getting over one phase of treatment and preparing for the next.

I also appreciate that not all women are fortunate enough to be in my situation, with a large slab of paid time off work, a supportive partner and no dependent children. Any woman who can manage her cancer treatment while holding down a job and bringing up a family, especially as a sole parent, deserves to be bowed down to—although I'm sure she'd rather have an all-expenses-paid holiday in a five-star resort with built-in babysitter and masseuse.

The reason for the bone density scan is that my oncologist has recommended that I take Arimidex, an aromatase inhibitor, for five years after my radiation. My breast cancer is hormone-receptor positive, which is the case for over 50% of breast cancers. It means that my hormones, namely estrogen, stimulate the growth of cancer cells. Aromatase inhibitors prevent the estrogen from feeding the cancer cells, thereby minimising the risk of the cancer recurring, but one of their side-effects can be a loss of bone density. A bone density scan will provide a base level of measurement to track any loss.

I fully expect to have an A+ on my bone density report card. After all, I eat well, take calcium supplements and exercise regularly, including working out in the gym with weights. Not to mention the A pluses I already have for my post-op physiotherapy assessment and my report from the lymphedema clinic (no sign of lymphedema and the risk of it occurring being minimal).

Obviously I've forgotten the lesson from *Embracing Uncertainty* on letting go of expectations. The results come back that I have osteoporosis. This is a condition in which the bones become brittle and fragile due to the loss of bone density and are more susceptible to fractures. It's more common in older people, particularly women; and poor diet, excessive drinking, smoking and lack of exercise are risk factors.

'How can that be?' I demand of my doctor. 'I'm the healthiest person I know.'

He shrugs, kindly ignoring the irony of my statement. 'You have a small frame and you're thin, they're risk factors. And there may be an hereditary factor.'

I know that my mother (who has passed away) was never diagnosed with osteoporosis and neither has my father. But people often don't know they have it until they have a fracture and undergo an X-ray or scan.

'And I'm too young to have it,' I added. I've always associated osteoporosis with bent-over old ladies with dowager's humps.

But you can only be in denial for so long, and Dr Google informs me that an estimated 66% of Australia's over-50 population have osteoporosis or the forerunner to it, osteopenia. That makes me feel marginally better. My doctor's advice is to continue my current lifestyle and my bone density will be monitored to track if there's any loss, with medication adjustment if needed.

While I'm waiting to begin my radiation treatment, two important things happen. Firstly, as my sick leave from work is due to expire shortly, I submit my resignation. Even though this has been the plan all along, I still feel a few flutters of trepidation. It's a big move to give up a regular and secure source of income even though I have enough money coming in to replace it. But I focus on the positive things that are already coming from it and will continue to come from it.

Despite my constant interruptions for medical appointments and procedures, I've already achieved so much more with my writing than if I'd continued working. And my writing routine has given structure to my days and helped keep me sane in those difficult times of waiting for test results, and the occasional down times of feeling out of sorts and unmotivated. Forcing myself to write at those times has always made me feel more uplifted.

The second important thing is an email I receive from Breast Cancer Network Australia with the subject title *Robin – we dare you!* It's referring to their Skydive Challenge inviting members to participate in a free skydive on 14 February next year (2016), in return for raising a minimum of $2500 for the organisation.

As I stare at those words, it seems as if they're directed at me personally—that somehow they have divined that I'm chicken when it comes to activities of physical daring and that every time the subject of skydiving comes up in conversation, I've always said, 'You'll never catch me jumping out of a plane!'

And furthermore, those words know that I hate small planes and am so prone to motion sickness that I've been known to make myself nauseous on a children's swing. But regardless, they're taunting me. 'Come on, we dare you! Get out of your comfort zone!'

So I sign up for the Skydive Challenge straight away before I can change my mind. Once my official donation page is set up, I start hitting up friends and family for donations. Their reactions range from disbelief—'You? Jumping out of a plane?'; to grudging admiration—'Glad it's you and not me'; and to envy—'I've always wanted to do that!'

I do have an ulterior motive—I'm thinking that my skydive will make a great final chapter for this book, an excellent way to end it on a high note. Because this is not something I would ever have considered if I hadn't had breast cancer.

And I do wonder, in my more rational moments, what I've let myself in for. But it's only September now; so it's five months away, comfortably far enough into the future that I can put it out of my mind. As I've said before, sometimes procrastination is your best friend.

*

On my first day of radiation therapy, I turn up at the oncology clinic at the appointed time. This is another reason that I'm so fortunate—there is only one radiation clinic in my entire region and I happen to live only five minutes drive away. I'm issued with a swipe ID card and a seersucker gown, which could have been a tablecloth in a former life, and sit in the waiting room after changing into it.

After I'm called into the treatment room, I lie topless on the bed with my arms above my head, the other breast modestly covered up while the two therapists check my measurements and radiation doses. It takes some time, and I'm getting pins and needles in my arms.

'We only have to do this checking for the first time,' they assure me. 'Next time will be a lot quicker.' There's a mural on the ceiling of a vividly blue, cloud-flecked sky and another of a colourful flowering shrub, no doubt designed to make me feel cheerful, which they do.

When the therapists have finished measuring, they disappear into the control room. It's a weird sensation lying alone in a large room with this space age-like machine looming beside me. A red light near the doorway signals that the radiation beam is on and I half expect someone to announce, 'Mission control, ready for take-off!' and to be ejected into the bright blue sky on the ceiling mural.

I lie perfectly still, as instructed, as the machine moves around me. I can't feel the radiation beam but I imagine it working like a ray gun, shooting down the cancer cells as soon as they pop their little heads up. I find out the truth later—that radiation kills all the cells, good and bad, but the dose is low enough that the good cells can regenerate and the bad ones can't. Nonetheless, my Star Wars-like scenario of the rays fighting the evil cells is a comforting one.

This is the process every weekday for the next four weeks. Each Friday I receive my schedule for the next week, as my appointment times are different each day. I soon feel like a member of an exclusive club as I march in the front door daily with the confidence born of familiarity, greet the receptionist, swipe my ID card, and go inside to change into my gown and sit in the waiting room.

As I'm waiting, I surreptitiously eye my fellow members of the Radiotherapy VIP Club, wondering what they're here for. As breast and prostate cancer are two of the most common cancers treated by radiation, I assume that's the diagnosis for many of them. I'm frequently called into the treatment room straight away and rarely have to wait for longer than five minutes, so I never have time to indulge in more than a smile and a 'hello'.

The radiation sessions are short—less than five minutes from the time I'm called into the treatment room. I soon come to the conclusion that out of all the professions, radiation therapists derive the highest job satisfaction. As they're making sure my body is positioned correctly, with one making adjustments and the other reading the computer screen, there's a constant flow of superlatives. 'Beautiful!' 'Terrific!' 'Fantastic!'

I'm gratified that in some small way I've contributed to that satisfaction.

In line with my resolve to take advantage of everything that's offered to me, I attend a couple of information sessions run by the oncology clinic. The first is called *Beating Cancer With Food and Exercise.* Being the health nut I am, I already know most of the information.

One of the issues discussed was, does a diet high in sugar contribute to cancer? Scientific theory is divided on this issue—some experts say there is a clear link between excessive sugar and cancer while others say it is only when that sugar intake leads to high blood sugar, diabetes and obesity that it's a risk. The nutritionist running the information sessions discusses all these points of view but, interestingly, doesn't answer the question.

I've been following the Paleo regime for some time (modified—I eat cheese and yoghurt to maintain my calcium levels) as I find it works well for my digestive issues. One of their tenets is to give up processed foods, including processed sugar, and to use natural sugars (coconut sugar, raw honey, pure maple syrup) sparingly.

Prior to my cancer diagnosis, I allowed myself an occasional indulgence of a small amount of dark chocolate, my favourite treat, two or three times a week, but have over the last few months given that up as well. It's amazing how you don't miss sweet things once you're used to not having them and your tastebuds adjust accordingly.

I can also understand why sugar is being touted as an addiction on the same level as heroin. On the couple of occasions recently when I've relented and treated myself to some chocolate (when I've been in a low mood), my tastebuds have gone into ecstasy overload as soon as the sweetness hits them. I literally get a high from chocolate! However, the good thing is that because the taste is so intense, I only need a small amount, two to four squares, to feel satisfied.

The second information session, two weeks into my treatment, is on radiotherapy and how it works. One of the issues discussed is side-effects; and one of the advantages of radiotherapy is that unlike chemotherapy, it has few side effects. The main ones are fatigue and burning, similar to sunburn, in the affected area.

I have felt the occasional strong desire to go for a nap in the middle of the day, which is not surprising when I consider all that activity that's going on inside me—all those cells being mowed down and the good ones getting up, shaking themselves off and concentrating on growing again.

I haven't experienced any burning yet, but I'm informed it often doesn't occur until the third week and may continue for a couple of weeks after treatment. From all accounts, it's a painful experience; so from the next week on, I wake up every morning wondering if today will be the day I start to get the burns. But no burning occurs right up until my last day of treatment.

There's a tradition at the oncology clinic that on their last day, patients can, if they choose, place their painted handprint on the 'wall of fame', to celebrate the end of their treatment. I choose bright pink, the nurse slaps the paint all over my hand and I find a space down at the bottom of the wall, which is already jostling with handprints of every size and colour.

Looking at the handprints of all those people who have come and gone before me, I wonder where they all are now. Was their treatment successful and are they back to normality, whatever that means for them? Or have they encountered further obstacles? I'm only one of so many; it's a bittersweet feeling of both hope and sadness. But I don't have time to contemplate the greater questions of the universe as it's Friday and I'm off to Brisbane for the weekend, for a writers' conference. I had booked and paid for it months ago, estimating I'd probably be finished with my treatment by this time. My calculations were spot-on and it's a wonderful way to celebrate.

On the way, I stop into a chemist and pick up some MooGoo, recommended as the best cream to soothe radiation burns. It's just a precaution in case they happen—I don't want my weekend to be spoiled by feeling as if my chest is on fire. The history of MooGoo is interesting—— apparently it was first used to heal cows' udders and keep them in good condition for milking.

Because it was full of so many natural and effective skincare ingredients, it was adapted for human use, not only for radiation burns but also as an all-round moisturiser.

I wonder who had the bright idea of using it for humans? Perhaps one fine day, a milkmaid, as she rubbed some MooGoo onto her cow's cracked teats, had an epiphany.

'My poor old nipples are a bit dry, the westerlies just whip straight through this muslin and my breasts could do with a bit of tender loving care.' She looked around surreptitiously, unbuttoned the top half of her pinafore and smothered her breasts in goo.

She soon got into a routine—'one for the cow, one for me'— and it wasn't long before the other milkmaids in the servants' quarters noticed her beautifully soft chest as they were all having their weekly sponge baths. They begged her to tell them her secret, so she did, and they all started pilfering large quantities of MooGoo and rubbing it all over themselves. The rest is history. (Except for the poor dairy farm owner who wondered why he was constantly running out of MooGoo).

I don't end up using the MooGoo, nor do I experience any burning at the conference or afterwards. At my follow-up appointment with my radiation oncologist a couple of weeks later, I mention this.

'You're one of the lucky ones,' she says. 'It's usually the more well-endowed ladies who experience it.'

Another reason, if I needed any more, to be modestly endowed.

What Next?

It's December. I relax and coast into Christmas. Usually at this time of year, I experience end-of-year burnout—depression, irritability and fatigue. It's as if I can shoulder the load of my busy life for 11 months of the year then come December, my body decides it's had enough and goes on strike. But for the first time in years I have no burnout. It's a wonderful feeling.

The relentless grind of treatment officially ended a month ago. All I have left is daily medication and six monthly check-ups. I have conflicting emotions; I feel light and free, like a bird that's been let out of a cage gliding along on the air currents. But I also feel a sense of anticlimax—my full-time job as breast cancer patient is over, leaving a gap in my life, albeit a welcome gap.

This is a very normal emotion. There's a certain comfort in having a team of experts looking after you, constantly monitoring your wellbeing. When it's over, people often feel vulnerable, wondering, 'Who's looking after me now?' Others will stop asking you how you are because they know your treatment's over and you look well, and friends and family expect you to be back to normal and to carry on with your life.

But slotting back into your normal life is not so easy. For a start, it often takes your body months, even years, to recover from the after-effects of chemotherapy and radiation, (eg, fatigue and 'chemobrain'—problems with memory and inability to focus) and you may be dealing with ongoing issues such as lymphedema, early menopause and the side effects of hormone medication.

Then there are the psychological challenges. Author Margaret Lesh, in her book *Let Me Get This Off My Chest*, writes about preparing to go back to her job as a court reporter after treatment for breast cancer.

'What I found during that time (she was off work) was that the physical recovery was maybe half; the other half was mental. I had to overcome my fear of moving on. Really there were a multitude of fears—the fear of going back into the world, of having this invisible sign hanging around my neck that read, "this person had breast cancer."'

Returning to a familiar job she knew inside out and colleagues she'd known for years suddenly seemed scary. 'Attorneys I'd known for years had no idea what I'd been through. It felt odd, almost like I was hiding this big secret. A big secret that had absolutely no effect on the way I was able to perform my job, but somehow I just felt different.'

Even though I didn't return to my previous job, I have experienced those same feelings of having a sign around my neck saying, 'I've had breast cancer'. It's a feeling common to those who've been through a traumatic experience—like a prisoner thinking they have 'jailbird' tattooed on their forehead once they're back out in the community. It's because the experience we've been through is so embedded in our psyche that we think others can see it too; when the reality is that we look perfectly ordinary to everyone else.

And Margaret found once she returned to work that she wasn't alone. During a break in a court hearing, she overheard one of the expert witnesses talking about how he'd been on leave for prostate cancer. She confided in him about her own cancer experience and says, 'The man's demeanour changed instantly. We were part of the club—the club no one wants to be a member of. We swapped stories and I watched him choke up while telling me about his journey.'

Margaret also discovered during a conversation with the judge, a young female, that she had also had breast cancer, and had undergone a mastectomy and chemotherapy. They hugged, no longer strangers. As she says, 'survivors are everywhere'.

And a significant percentage of those survivors would have experienced a common after-effect of cancer treatment—depression. During treatment, we're so busy with our medical regime and holding it all together that it's often not till we have finished our treatment that we're able to fully come to terms with our diagnosis.

Sometimes this delayed effect hits hard. Cindy, whom I met at the oncology clinic, told me she went through a lumpectomy, removal of lymph nodes and a harrowing round of chemo (causing her husband to nickname her 'Chemo Bitch'). She then had to attend a number of weeks of radiotherapy. She emerged from her first session bawling like a baby.

'What's wrong?' her husband asked, alarmed and no doubt thinking, 'What did they do to her in there?'

'I've got cancer,' she sobbed. Months after her initial diagnosis, it had only just sunk in.

Anxiety often goes hand in hand with depression. Anxiety about the uncertainty of the future, what the next stage of life will bring, how we will cope. Then there's the fear of the cancer returning. Although this fear can diminish with time, it never completely goes away. Cancer survivors of ten, even twenty years and more say they still get anxious when it's time for their check-up or mammogram and breathe a sigh of relief when they get the all-clear.

That anxiety can also surface if you hear of others' cancer returning. There are many cases of cancer survivors being clear for years then being diagnosed with another bout of breast cancer or, worse, secondary cancer, for which there is no cure.

I have read articles claiming that there's a 30% chance of breast cancer survivors being later diagnosed with secondary breast cancer, regardless of whether you had an early diagnosis and how many years you've been clear. That's a scary statistic and I think about my surgeon Scott's reassurance that I will be cured. Can anyone ever say they're cured?

Regardless of this possible prognosis, I don't want to live my life in constant fear of my cancer recurring. In a philosophical sense, this is not something I have any control over. I will do everything in my power to maintain my health with good diet, exercise, relaxation and a positive attitude; but sometimes even all those things are not enough. However, being fearful and anxious will not stop the cancer recurring if that is what it's destined to do.

I think about my friend Kay, whose cancer reappeared in the same breast after 15 years in the clear. I know she wasn't sitting around wondering if the cancer was going to come back and bite her—she got on with her life. And I'll do the same.

I find the practice of mindfulness very effective in dealing with this fear—or any fears for that matter. Mindfulness is an ancient practice found in a range of Eastern philosophies such as yoga and Buddhism. It's often a part of meditation, but you don't have to meditate to be mindful. Mindfulness is about focusing your awareness in the present moment and being aware of your thoughts, feelings and bodily sensations without judgment.

Over time you develop the capacity to mentally step outside of yourself and observe your thoughts and feelings without getting caught up in them, which then means you have more control over them. It means you're not reacting instantaneously to things that happen to you or are said to you; instead, you're able to pause and make a conscious decision on how you will respond.

For example, when I think about my cancer coming back and feel that constriction of anxiety in my chest, I say to myself, 'I am experiencing fear of my cancer returning. This is not serving any useful purpose and I don't want to be fearful, so I will now replace that thought with another more positive thought.'

Like anything, it takes practice. For more information and tips on mindfulness, check out Leo Baubata's blog *Zen Habits*. He has also published some excellent books on the subject, which are listed on his website. There is also a wide variety of relaxation and mindfulness exercises on *YouTube*.

The bottom line is that some women suffering post-treatment depression are in a deep hole and feel incapable of shaking off the 'black dog'. If that's you, I implore you to seek help from your doctor, your local cancer help organisation or any other counselling agency; there are many people who are willing and able to help you.

On a happier note, the one outcome of a breast cancer diagnosis that is common to most women is that it forces you to stop in your tracks and reassess your life. Dr Rachel Nemen, an oncologist and author of the bestselling book *Kitchen Table Wisdom: Stories That Heal*, says our identities are wrapped up in our day-to-day lives.

'Often, we espouse values that are unexamined—we do things out of habit and not out of conviction. When cancer comes, we're no longer able to fulfil those roles and we're stripped of what we do. Cancer can shuffle our values like a deck of cards. Sometimes the card we carried at the bottom of our deck turns out to be the top card, the thing that really matters.'

Many women not only take the opportunity to reassess their lives but also take on a whole new direction—maybe something they've always wanted to do but for many reasons have held themselves back, as in my case of becoming a full-time author. Or perhaps it's something they've never considered, but their diagnosis of breast cancer and the realisation of their own mortality has made them much more open to new experiences.

Psychologist Florence Strang started her blog *100 Perks of Having Cancer* after being diagnosed with breast cancer; not as a way of making light of it but as a means of staying positive through her treatment of mastectomy, chemotherapy and radiation. Each post was about a different perk she had discovered, many of them humorous (eg, I didn't have to wax my upper lip, I didn't have to worry about my guests finding a hair in the food) and she readily admits that finding 100 good things about cancer was no easy task. She continues the blog now that she has finished her treatment, and, with co-author Susan Gonzalez, she turned the blog into the book *100 Perks of Having Cancer plus 100 Health Tips For Surviving It.*

Florence credits the blog with changing her life. In the book, she says, 'Blogging not only provided me with a great distraction from my illness but it also gave me a positive and creative outlet for my feelings. Writing my blog and now this book has been one of the most therapeutic perks of having cancer.'

Stories of women changing careers and finding a whole new lifestyle after breast cancer are common. Katie, who has survived two bouts of breast cancer and a bilateral mastectomy, was an audiologist working 45 hours a week before her diagnosis, with little time or energy for anything else. After her first diagnosis, she moved from the city to a small town with a creative and spiritual community, and became a massage therapist. After her second diagnosis seven years later, she decided to explore her creativity and moved into web design, jewellery making, choir singing and photography. 'It pushed me to explore my spirituality and my personal development.'

Sometimes you don't have a choice about returning to your previous job; your health precludes it. Rochelle was working as a flight attendant before she was diagnosed with breast cancer and at the age of 32 had a bilateral mastectomy. Afterwards, she went back to her job but soon realised she couldn't maintain the lifestyle.

In a post on her blog *Cancer Triathlon*, she writes, 'During the 14+ months of treatment, I was introduced to a new way of living, a way of living I had given up in my early 20s. A day that consisted of meals at appropriate mealtimes and routine. And I loved it. To return to flying and have my body forced into different time zones and eating patterns has been a challenge. A challenge I no longer feel I can continue with. A challenge that has become a struggle.'

So, making her health a priority, she resigned from QANTAS after nearly 10 years of service and has found her 'new normal' undertaking a full-time university course.

Taking new directions, as I said previously, is due in no small part to the realisation of our own mortality. As we go about our normal daily lives, the knowledge is there in the back of our minds that we'll depart this earth one day; but we avoid thinking about it because it's too scary or depressing. Especially when we're in our twenties and thirties—death is so far into the future that we rarely give it a thought. But the older we get, the more often we're confronted with it—our parents and other relatives die, then our peers. I had two friends the same age as me die of cancer in their fifties, which made me really take stock of my life.

But even so, the awareness of our own death is often still an intellectual process. Let's face it, when a friend or relative is diagnosed with a life-threatening illness, much as it is distressing for us, deep down we think, 'I'm glad it's not me.'

But then we get the diagnosis of breast cancer and it *is* us; and the fact that we're going to die, at some point, hits us hard right in our emotional core. Even those of us with early breast cancer and a good prognosis don't escape it. What if we hadn't been diagnosed early? What if the mammogram hadn't picked up the lump? What if it had been a very aggressive cancer? There are so many 'what-ifs' that you can drive yourself crazy thinking about them; but the fact remains that we've had, at the very least, a glimpse of our own ending and at most, a brush with death. This is a powerful incentive to think about what we really want out of life and go for it.

And a glimpse of your own ending is not something you want to dwell on. A few years ago I attended the funeral of a friend

who had died of a brain tumour at 53. The church was packed;
people were standing in the aisles and spilling out all the doors.
Anxiety gripped me. No way would I have this many people
attending my funeral – I'd be lucky to fill a quarter of the
church. (Not that I'm a horrible person, you understand; I just
don't have a very wide circle of friends). Was the number of
people who attended your funeral a measure of your life's worth,
and the impact you had had on the world? If so, I had some
serious work ahead of me. I needed to embark on a campaign to
be more sociable and make new friends; ie going out more,
maybe joining a few clubs, doing more at-home entertaining.

Then, having made these new friends, I'd have to keep in regular contact. Friends you've known for years (which comprise a
good part of my social circle) don't care if you only phone them
once every three months, but new friendships require much more
maintenance. ('Robin who? I only met her a couple of times. She
died? I won't bother going to her funeral').

The whole process of planning a jam-packed funeral sounded
much too exhausting and time-consuming. Okay, I know what
you're thinking – 'You won't care when you're dead!' Of course I
was aware of that all along, but that just illustrates the irrational
nature of our emotions. In the end I decided that the stress of
making and keeping new friendships would probably lead to my
early demise, which would be tragic if I hadn't achieved my goal
of 100 new friends, and if it looked as if attendees at my funeral
might be a bit light on, the organisers could always hire profes-
sional mourners.

Back to living. Part of the process of reassessment of our
lives, as oncologist Rachel Nemen says, entails realising what's
important to us and what we may have been neglecting. 'Stop
and smell the roses,' 'Don't sweat the small stuff,' 'Live every
minute as if it's your last.' All of these clichés are trotted out by
people who've been diagnosed with a serious illness, and just
because they're clichés doesn't make them any less real or true.
Clichés are born of truth; but because they are so overused, they

lose their impact. However, for the people who experience those feelings, it's as if they are discovering them for the first time; and if you haven't been there yourself, they're just glib phrases.

Says Rochelle, 'I've changed in character—when something is taken away from you, you really learn how to focus.' She has a more relaxed attitude now; things still upset her but she can let go of them quickly. 'You learn how to roll with the punches and have to be able to see the humour. If you don't laugh, you cry; and I've never been much of a crier.'

'I've become more fatalistic,' Katie says. 'Shit happens and you just have to deal with it.'

Blogger Hilene Flanzbaum, in an article *The Possibility of Joy: How Breast Cancer Changed My Life* says, 'I noticed that I was noticing my life. It was as if someone had stood next to me in the supermarket line and yelled in my ear, in the loudest voice imaginable—"Wake up!!!!" I stopped sleepwalking through my days. I started paying attention. I won't say clichéd things like "colours seemed brighter" or "flowers smelled sweeter". I am not sure they did. I just felt a new sense grow in me—I became conscious of time; I was alert in a new way. I felt things more deeply.'

I can relate to her statement about paying more attention to my surroundings. I often pause to take in where I am—the sights, sounds and smells—and what I'm doing. It's a part of learning to appreciate your life as it is right now, not how you'd like it to be—another aspect of mindfulness. However, I do find it a challenge as my tendency is to live in my head, thinking about story ideas, plots and characters—an occupational hazard of being an author. You have to be able to block out your surroundings to write, and when I'm in the flow, an atomic bomb could hit and I'd be none the wiser. Consequently, I'm also good at zoning out and daydreaming when I'm not writing and admittedly, my best ideas often come to me then. So that's my excuse for not always succeeding in being in the present moment, but I'm improving.

I also cope better with uncertainty, and don't feel so anxious and fearful about things that are outside of my control. I have also learnt not to invest so much in expectations and following Susan Jeffers' recommendations mentioned earlier, I try to keep an open mind and to wonder rather than hope.

As for not sweating the small stuff, which is often cited as a positive outcome of cancer, that's a lesson in progress for me. I'm one of those people who can cope with major adversity but get frustrated with small annoyances, like my computer freezing or not being able to find my car keys. But I'm working on it and this is an area where mindfulness can help—developing the ability to pause and calm myself before the frustration builds up.

Relationships are another part of our lives that come to the fore with a breast cancer diagnosis. We often take our relationships for granted in the rush and bustle of daily living, and every woman I spoke to said that their cancer diagnosis brought home to them how much love and support they had from family and friends. As one survivor said, 'It's a shame that it takes this to realise how much your friends and family love you and will be there for you.'

This was certainly the case with me—I was grateful on many occasions (and still am) for the love of Aaron, my children and other family members and friends. I can't begin to imagine what it would be like coping with this experience alone.

Another outcome for me is that I have occasionally experienced bouts of survivors' guilt. I am very conscious of how lucky I am to have been diagnosed early and not lost my breast or undergone chemo as I know many women who've undergone those experiences and more. It has been especially brought home to me while researching this book, reading numerous stories of the trauma suffered by women in various stages of treatment. It seems that Fate deals the cards of survivorship in a haphazard and illogical way. Women who are given a poor prognosis can survive for decades, and those who have sailed through their treatment and are given the all clear, can end up losing the battle. It really seems like the luck of the draw, which contributes to those thoughts of guilt. 'How come I'm so lucky? Why them? Why not me?'

Wendy Harpham, a doctor who is in her 25th year of survivorship, has written a very perceptive article *Guilty*, for the *Oncology Times*. She writes about a friend, Ellen, also diagnosed with breast cancer, whom she met early on in her treatment, and who subsequently died. Wendy felt guilty about all the milestones in her life that she was enjoying that Ellen couldn't, until she realized that guilt was not serving any useful purpose. 'Survivor's guilt is good when it energizes people in life-enhancing ways,' she says. 'But guilt becomes a problem when all it does is make people feel miserable, keeping them from enjoying life's blessings.'

Furthermore, she knew that if Ellen were privy to her feelings of guilt, she would be angry with Wendy for allowing them to spoil her good fortune. Wendy concludes the article with, 'But I never allow myself the luxury of feeling guilty about my good fortune because the most powerful way for me to honour Ellen's memory is to delight wholeheartedly in all that is right in my world.'

I think that's a great way to view survivorship and I have adopted that attitude myself. If I find myself feeling guilty for my good fortune, I quickly change my attitude to one of appreciation and gratitude.

If you'd like to read more about life after treatment, check out the Resources page at the back where I've listed some articles and videos.

Laugh And The World Laughs With You

Laughter is the best medicine. Another cliché, but nevertheless it contains a lot of truth. The role of humour in recovery from illness has been well researched and documented.

The most famous example is that of Norman Cousins, who was diagnosed in the 1960s with a crippling degenerative disease called ankylosing spondylitis. After suffering adverse reactions to his medication and having read about the power of positive emotions, he decided to take matters into his own hands. He checked out of the hospital and into a hotel, set up a movie projector in his room and began a daily regimen of massive Vitamin C doses and a constant stream of humorous shows, mainly Marx Brothers movies and episodes of Candid Camera. He claimed that ten minutes of belly laughs while watching Groucho Marx before bed afforded him an extra two hours of pain-free sleep. Groucho Marx himself said, 'A clown is like an aspirin, only he works twice as fast.'

Cousins' symptoms gradually disappeared and he made an almost complete recovery. He then went on to help establish a department at the University of California to investigate the connection between illness and the mind. He continued to laugh frequently until his death at 75, living many years longer than doctors predicted.

Many medical experts are dubious about his claim that laughter and vitamins had cured his illness. There is some doubt that his original diagnosis was correct, and some say that his recovery was a natural process that would have happened anyway, regardless of his treatment.

To me, the moral of the story is: Just because science hasn't proved that laughter can cure illness, or even contribute to a cure, doesn't mean it isn't true. And there is certainly evidence to support the notion that laughter elevates pain thresholds, reduces stress, boosts immunity and enhances quality of life. Who wouldn't want less pain and stress, and more joy in their lives? Especially when undergoing treatment for cancer.

Humour is often used as a complementary cancer therapy in hospitals and other treatment agencies. Many offer humorous books and DVDs for patients and clown visits to hospitals are widely embraced, by both children and adults.

Many facilities run group laughter therapy sessions, which are not based on humour or jokes but on laughter as a physical exercise. For example, one exercise involves participants standing in a circle, putting their fingers on their cheekbones, chest or abdomen and making 'ha ha' or 'he he' sounds until they feel the vibrations in their body. The laughter soon becomes contagious and it's hard for others not to join in.

Laughter yoga, developed by Indian physician Madan Kataria, operates on a similar basis. I attended a laughter yoga session many years ago as research for an article I was writing. The exercises were similar to the one above, and we also did laughter greetings and fake laughter—the idea being that fake laughter soon becomes real laughter.

I felt very self-conscious, which is normal for a first-timer; and even though I did laugh, it felt forced. I think I would have gained more benefit, and certainly more genuine laughter, from watching one of my favourite Monty Python sketches. However, don't let that put you off if you want to try it. Many people swear by laughter groups/yoga (in between giggling and guffawing) and I concede that I formed an opinion based on one session. I'm sure it takes a few sessions, for some people at least, to relax and feel the benefits.

And I should qualify that reference to Monty Python. I'm an asthmatic and even though I rarely suffer serious asthma attacks, the one impact it does have on my life is that I get laughter-induced asthma. Whenever I laugh heartily, I end up in a fit of coughing, wheezing and spluttering; so for me, watching my favourite Monty Python sketches may not be so beneficial in the short term. But I'm not going to stop enjoying them, or anyone else who makes me laugh, so I'm hoping the long-term benefits will outweigh any short-term discomfort.

Once you start searching for it, you'll find a lot of humour about breast cancer on the internet. Even Google itself has a sense of humour—of sorts—when it comes to cancer. While researching humorous breast cancer stories, one of the 'searches related to' suggestions at the bottom of the page said 'fun facts about breast cancer'.

'How intriguing,' I thought and, always eager to catch up on any fun I might have missed, I clicked on the link. But not one site came up with any fun facts. There were plenty of facts, enough to make your head spin, but none that remotely resembled fun. Perhaps this was Google's idea of fun, sending me on a wild goose chase.

I suspect that 'fun facts about' is a generic searching suggestion and that if you were to google 'being eaten alive by deadly tarantulas', there would be a search suggestion saying 'fun facts about being eaten alive by deadly tarantulas'.

While I was on that page searching in vain for fun facts about breast cancer, the 'searches related to' suggestions at the bottom of the page changed tone to 'shocking facts about breast cancer' and 'how many people die of breast cancer every year'. Now I knew for sure that Google was messing with my mind. Needless to say, I didn't click on the links. In this instance, ignorance is bliss!

One of the gems I did find was the article *Ask the Mutant: Take Two Limericks and Call Me in the Morning* by Eva Moon. Eva discovered she carried the BRCA genetic mutation, of which the risk of breast cancer is 85% and ovarian cancer is 50%. The recommended preventative action is surgery—a hysterectomy and bilateral mastectomy.

So she did the only sensible, rational thing when you find out you're going to lose a large percentage of your female parts. She wrote a limerick:

I've just had a genetic test
And I'm feeling a little depressed
It's not just because
I'll have menopause
But I wasn't quite done with my breasts

She posted it on the forum of *FORCE* website—*Facing Our Risk Of Cancer Empowered*, a non-profit organisation for women with high heredity breast and ovarian cancer risk. It struck a chord with other members; and over the next few months, women all over the world wrote hundreds of limericks and posted them on the forum.

'No subject was off-limits,' Eva says in the article. 'We rhymed about our genes, families, husbands, lost loved ones, nail-biting waits for test results, mammograms, approaching surgery dates, protracted recoveries, flagging libidos and constipation. These were the people who understood when no one else in our lives did. And along the way, we became friends.'

Eva herself didn't stop at one—she wrote limericks about each step of the way as she underwent her surgeries and recovery. Here's another one:

On the couch 'cause my legs are like jelly
Watching old flicks on the telly
Hysterectomy's done
And it sure isn't fun
When the cat wants to walk on my belly

Eva associates limericks with childhood and laughter, and I can certainly relate to that. As children, my two brothers and I often made up limericks on long car journeys—it made a welcome break from 'I Spy', and the endless and monotonous 'Are we there yet?'

It was even more fun when we took it in turns to make up a line. Warning: If playing this version of the game, you must make a rule that the person who makes up the first line must end it with a word that's easily rhymed with. This rule was set in stone after many backseat car fights after the beginner deliberately ended the first line with words like 'orange', 'purple' or 'wolf'.

I couldn't resist the challenge, so here's mine:

Well-endowed I'm definitely not
But I'm happy with what I've got
A little less breast
And a scar east to west
But to my man I'll always be hot.

Try it yourself. At worst, you'll spend a couple of hours having fun (or eliminate limerick-writing forever from your bucket list) and at best, you'll discover a talent you didn't know you had!

And most importantly, humour is the most fun when it's shared. Laughter is contagious and things are often funnier when you're with others. It's why you'll invariably find that a comedy movie is funnier when you see it at the cinema than if you see it alone at home. There's something very basically human and connecting about laughing together. As humourist and musician Victor Borge said, 'Laughter is the shortest distance between two people.' Perhaps if we put all the warring factions in the world into cinemas and made them sit through a marathon of funny movies, we'd have world peace—for a few hours, at least.

If you'd like to explore more humorous articles or videos on breast cancer, check out the Resources page at the back. And if you fancy a bit of beefcake with your humour, there's a free Your Man Reminder app for smart phones in which well-built, bare-chested guys show you how to do breast examinations and remind you daily. There's also an amusing video about the app on *YouTube*.

I guess that's the next best thing to having a hunky guy in your bedroom giving you a hands-on demonstration. But wait— I have!

A hunky guy, anyway, which is a start. After I was diagnosed, a couple of people joked that I should blame Aaron for not examining my breasts thoroughly enough and finding the lump before the mammogram did. I won't go that far but that's one more chore I can delegate to him.

AARON'S LIST OF THINGS TO DO

Take out garbage
Wash car
De-cobweb the garage
Feel my breasts

The Last Laugh

With breast cancer, the elephant in the room is always, 'What if it comes back? What if I get secondary breast cancer and die?'

Or perhaps you've already been diagnosed with secondary, also known as metastatic breast cancer, which means it has spread to other parts of the body. Although there is no cure, only treatment to alleviate symptoms, many women in this situation live for years after diagnosis. But they know there's an end date even if they don't know exactly when it is.

I can't even begin to think what that must be like so all my comments in this section will be based on what I've read, and my own observations of terminally ill friends and relatives. But I thought it was important for me to include this chapter, as some of you reading this book would have been diagnosed with secondary breast cancer and may be thinking, 'That's all very well that humour helps in the recovery from breast cancer, but I'm not going to recover.'

But, as you may have already discovered, humour plays an important role in enhancing the quality of your life. The average person could be forgiven for thinking that those with a terminal illness would find little to laugh about. However, studies have shown that the reverse is true; they are often more likely to joke and laugh. The benefits of laughter during cancer treatment—elevation of pain thresholds, boosting immunity, reducing stress and connecting with others—are even more important when you know your time is limited. You want to make the most of the life you have left.

In an article for *Daily Mail: The Best Way to Cope with Cancer? Treat It As a Joke*, writer Lindsay Nicholson, whose husband and daughter both died of cancer before she was diagnosed with breast cancer, says, 'In my experience of cancer, sadly now quite extensive, it's always those who have endured the most tragedy and devastation who take greatest delight in sending up their situation.'

Further on she says, 'While it is often said that humour is tragedy after sufficient time has passed, a terminal diagnosis means that time must necessarily be telescoped and everything gets rolled into one, until you don't know whether you are weeping tears of laughter, or grief, or both.'

Some people are appalled when they hear someone who is dying cracking jokes about their own death. But in these instances, humour serves a number of important purposes—it's an expression of the person's feelings; a way of dealing with the fear and uncertainty; a need for closeness with others by making them laugh; and a way of feeling normal and forgetting about their illness, even if just for a few moments.

Any discomfort felt by onlookers is usually due to their own anxieties and fears about death. Being with a terminally ill person is very confronting as it forces us to think about our own demise. Even writing and researching this chapter has been confronting for me as I can't help but think about the possibility of this happening to me and how I would react. But from my own experiences of being with friends and relatives who are dying, they have welcomed and often instigated humour and laughter, which then has made it easier for me to reciprocate in kind.

The article *Humor and Oncology* in the *Journal of Clinical Oncology* says, 'It has been suggested that the use of humour permits patients to psychologically distance themselves from their own death, while still allowing an acknowledgment of their terminal condition, thus helping to limit their psychological level of awareness of their condition and being an acceptable way to deny reality.'

I love that—an acceptable way to deny reality. I'm an expert at denial (that's not a cobweb on the ceiling, I'm sure I could pass for forty, at a distance in a dim light) and I'm all for it if it makes life more bearable. That's why I'm a writer—so I can deny reality by living in my own fantasy world.

Women who joke in public about their imminent death are, in my opinion, particularly courageous. Advertising copywriter Fanny Gaynes wrote a book *How Am I Gonna Find a Man If I'm Dead?* She found humour in her situation despite the removal of both of her breasts, secondary breast cancer, and endless rounds of conventional and experimental treatments. She lived life to the full until she died in 1993, shortly before her book was published.

One of the best current examples is Nikki Martinez, nicknamed the Cancer Queen of Comedy. She was diagnosed with Stage 3 cancer in 2010 and had a mastectomy. 'I then decided to make cancer my career,' she says.

She performed her debut as a stand-up comedian in a breast cancer charity comedy show, which you can watch on *YouTube*, and has since developed a comedy routine around her diagnosis. She has performed all over the US, raising funds for breast cancer organisations and encouraging women to have regular mammograms. Even being diagnosed with secondary breast cancer in 2012 hasn't stopped her. If anything, it's increased her determination. She says she has a unique niche in the comedy world. 'You're not gonna find too many healthy women that're gonna whip off a wig and a fake boob, so that is probably the only advantage ... you can't really steal my jokes.'

She is positive that her sense of humour is keeping her alive. In an article *Beating Cancer with a Sense of Humor* she says, 'Laughter is the best medicine. If I cried as much as I laughed, I would have died a long time ago. Laughing is my way of giving it (cancer) the finger. I let cancer take my breast—not my life.'

Of course not everyone wants to become a comedian, but just finding the humour in everyday situations can be a great uplifter. The article *Humor and Oncology* also quotes this poignant comment from a terminally ill patient: 'The other reactions—anger, depression, suppression, denial—took a little piece of me with them. Each made me feel just a little less human. Laughter made me more open to ideas, more inviting to others and even a little stronger inside. It proved to me that, even as my body was devastated and my spirit challenged, I was still a vital human.'

That sums it up exactly. Humour is about humanity at its core. When we're laughing, we're not feeling sad, angry, lonely, frustrated, stressed or hard done by. We're joyful, in the here and now and connecting with others. Humankind at its best.

Ending On A
High Note

The day for my skydive has arrived. All week it's been rainy and windy; but the weather forecasters have been staunch in their prediction for a fine day today and for once they're right. The sun is smiling down upon us, ruffled by a light breeze.

I've raised $2600, just over the target of $2500. I held a movie night at my local cinema, which raised a few hundred dollars, and the rest has been through donations. As a result, I get to jump out of a plane entirely free of charge. It also happens to be 14 February, Valentine's Day.

When anyone asks me how I'm feeling about the big day, I say, 'What better way to spend Valentine's Day than floating through the clouds strapped up close and personal to a young, hunky skydiver?' (Of course I have no idea if my tandem jumper will be young and hunky; but if he's old and ugly, it wouldn't be much of a joke).

Up until today, I've tried not to think about it for two reasons. Firstly, I want to save all my emotional energy (including my fears and anxieties) for the day itself and secondly, it's damn scary. The times I do think about it, I use some cognitive behavioural therapy to re-frame my thoughts. *I'm not scared, I'm excited, I'm going to love it* and I visualise myself smiling from ear to ear as I'm floating to earth in the parachute.

Now as Aaron and I make the 45-minute journey to Red-cliffe, a coastal city on the northern outskirts of Brisbane where the jump is taking place, the reality of what I'm about to do sets in. My stomach starts churning. *Courage is being afraid but going ahead anyhow,* I remind myself. *I can do this.*

We arrive at the office of the skydive company and fill out the paperwork. I buy the full package of 150 photos and a five to seven minute video; I want to have as many mementos as I can of the experience. I meet the six other ladies who have also taken up the Be Brave for BCNA challenge and are taking the plunge. It's a national event—participants in three other states are also doing their skydive today.

Most of our group have had breast cancer and we exchange brief stories of our experiences. One woman has just been diag-nosed for a second time, receiving the news just before her five-year remission period was up. Another had a similar experience some time ago. Cancer is like a hardy weed—you think you've killed it but it just keeps popping up again.

All but one of us are skydive virgins and it's comforting to know that everybody else is feeling just as terrified as I am—even the one who's done it before. Cognitive behavioural thera-py be damned!

Aaron leaves to go the drop zone on nearby Bells Beach to await my landing, where my three children, my brother and a bottle of chilled champagne will also be waiting. BCNA have set up a celebration reception there for us and our supporters with lunch and a presentation ceremony.

We're then shepherded into the back room and given a brief spiel on what to expect. We'll be freefalling at up to 200 kilome-tres an hour for 50 seconds then parachuting for five to seven minutes. The freefall sounds terrifying—I've never done any-thing at 200 kilometres an hour. Due to my propensity for motion sickness, I've always avoided fast rides or vehicles or anything that looks dangerously sporty and speedy.

But there's no time to dwell on that as we're kitted up with our safety belts and harnesses, and introduced to our tandem partners. My partner Dave is neither young nor hunky, which is actually a relief—the not being young bit anyway. I figure if I'm going to be harnessed to a complete stranger as I'm jumping out of a plane, I want him to know what he's doing.

Dave gives me a rundown on what to do. 'Legs under the plane as we jump out then head back and legs up; then when I tap you on the shoulder, put your arms out to the side.'

How will I remember to do all those things when I'm busy being scared witless? We all file outside and board the bus that takes us to the airfield. The chatter around me is just background noise as I sit still and silent, taking slow, deep breaths. *Head back, legs up, arms out.* The 20-minute drive is over in five minutes, or so it seems.

We line up on a bench in front of the airfield and wait for our plane. Our tandem partners take group photos and videos, and get us shouting and smiling, like warm-up comedians before a live show. They will be wearing their tiny 'go pro' cameras strapped to their wrists during the skydive to take close-up photos and videos. Our plane taxis in and we board, waving bravely to the cameras. *Head back, legs up, arms out.*

We sit in pairs with our tandem partners on two bench seats that run the length of the plane. After waiting for clearance, we're finally off. The plane lurches into the air and we rise steadily to our destination of 10,000 feet. I took my motion sickness tablet earlier; but fortunately the ride is fairly smooth, so my stomach behaves itself.

Dave points out all the landmarks below. We're heading north to Bribie Island, about 57 kilometres away, where the plane will then turn around and we will jump out. It is indeed a spectacular view of mountains, beaches and towns, but I'm finding it hard to appreciate it. *Head back, legs up, arms out.*

Dave harnesses himself to me, and tightens my straps and

goggles. He turns on the camera and asks me how I'm feeling. 'A bit nervous,' I reply, a doyenne of understatement.

It only takes 15 minutes to reach our destination. It's time. The tandem partner at the head of the row opens the exit hatch. The wind roars in, icy cold. Now my heart is pumping—we're jumping out into that?

The first five jump out, one after the other. They're going so quickly—it's our turn already! *Head back, legs up, arms out.*

We slide over to the exit and before I can say 'Hold it, I've changed my mind', we're out. All I'm aware of is gusts of air rushing at my face and I'm finding it hard to breathe. I find out later in the photos that I have my eyes closed although I'm not aware of it at the time. My *head back, legs up, arms out* mantra has gone with the wind. Dave taps me on the shoulder and I obediently thrust my arms out in aeroplane position. And I needn't have worried about the speed of the freefall—to me it feels as if we're just floating in the one spot, like being suspended above a wind-blowing machine.

Then the parachute is up, we're vertical and I'm much more comfortable. Feeling more relaxed, I look around and take in the view below me—the neat patchwork of roads, houses and green fields, and the vast expanse of ocean. It's a strange feeling, being so high up and so exposed to the elements—just the two of us and all that sky and sea (apart from the six other parachutes, none of which I notice). 'You can let go of my arm now,' Dave says, although I wasn't aware I was holding his arm. Not so relaxed after all!

There are a couple of scary moments. Once we get caught in a gust of wind and shoot straight upwards. 'I think we might be going the wrong way,' I'm about to suggest to Dave and then we're heading downwards again. A few moments later we're spinning around in circles, and I'm pretty certain this isn't Dave performing party tricks with the parachute. My nervous yelp is blown away into the wind, but fortunately the spinning stops and we're coming in to land. I stick my legs out in front of me as instructed and we execute a perfect landing on the beach.

Dave helps me out of my harness. 'Would you do it again?' he asks. The camera's rolling. I laugh and shake my head with an emphatic 'No!'

After lots of hugs and kisses, and congratulations from the family, we crack open the champagne and have lunch. We sky-divers are presented with a certificate and a gift pack by the ladies from BCNA, more photos are taken and we each say a few words about the skydive and how we're feeling. We're all re-lieved that it's over, and elated that we conquered our fears and had an experience we'll never forget.

When it's my turn, I say, 'I would never have done this if I hadn't had breast cancer.' And it's true. If I hadn't been a mem-ber of BCNA, I wouldn't have received the email daring me to take up the challenge. And I'm so glad I did.

*

Over the next few days I'm still on a high. It's as much because I did something that was scary and out of character as the experi-ence itself. I can use this as a benchmark for any time in the future that I'm feeling afraid—is what I'm about to go through scarier than jumping out of a plane at 10,000 feet?

I watch the video several times to relive it—it was all over so quickly I hardly had time to process it. And contrary to my comment after I'd landed, I would do it again. I'm sure that next time I'd enjoy it even more, knowing what to expect. Will there be a next time? Who knows? The sky's the limit!

Finally ladies, a word of advice if you're thinking of doing a skydive. Forget about looking glamorous. Forget about even looking like your normal self. Tight goggles and gusts of air pounding your face at 200 kilometres an hour turn you into a caricature. In my case, with my nostrils flared like a thoroughbred racehorse and my top lip drawn back in a grimace to expose a mouthful of gums and teeth, I resembled a sure bet for the

Melbourne Cup.

But as we all know, looks count for very little when we're coping with breast cancer. Here's to health, happiness, and most of all, humour!

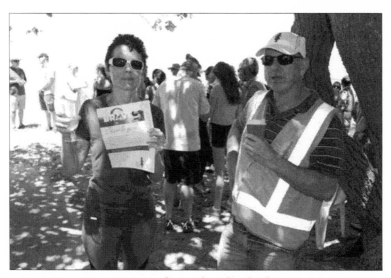

Aaron and me after the skydive

Resources

LIFE AFTER TREATMENT

Blogger Marie Ennis O'Connor talks about life after breast cancer treatment on her blog *Journey Beyond Breast Cancer* https://journeyingbeyondbreastcancer.com/ specifically aimed at helping women to cope after their treatment is over.

Her video about life after cancer is well worth watching. There is a link to it on the *About Me* page on her blog.

Alive With Joan https://alivewithjoan.com/#/?_k=g0g7fp a TV streaming network devoted to breast cancer issues, by well-known broadcaster and breast cancer survivor Joan Lunden.

An article in the *UK Telegraph: Life after Breast Cancer—Three Survivors'* *Stories.* http://www.telegraph.co.uk/lifestyle/9615701/Life-after-breast-cancer-three-survivors-stories.html

Blog post by marathon runner and blogger Nicki Miller *Two Years Later, Here Are 10 Ways Breast Cancer Changed Me.* http://womensrunning.competitor.com/2015/10/inspiration/two-years-later-here-are-10-ways-breast-cancer-changed-me_48073

The Best Breast Cancer Blogs of 2015. http://www.healthline.com/ health-slideshow/best-breast-cancer-blogs – A variety of blogs by women still undergoing treatment as well as post-treatment.

HUMOUR AND BREAST CANCER

Laughing in the Face of Cancer. http://www.laughingintheface ofcancer.com/

A blog started by Pam Lacko after she was diagnosed with ovarian cancer. She then discovered she had the BRCA genetic mutation, and had a preventative bilateral mastectomy. She has also written a book of the same name, available from the website.

Christine Clifford created *The Cancer Club* http://www.cancer club.com/ in 1995 in response to her experiences with breast cancer. In a short video on *YouTube,* https://www.youtube.com/ watch?v=0Lp3-XpFEQQ she reveals how she first discovered humour in cancer.

There are 20 humorous books on cancer listed on this blog post *Tackling Breast Cancer with Humour Books*: www.more.com /entertainment/books/tackling-breast-cancer-humor-books
Despite the title, these books cover a range of cancers but those on breast cancer include, 'Cancer Made Me A Shallower Person', 'Why I Wore Lipstick to My Mastectomy', '101 Uses For An Empty Bra' and 'Breastless in the City.'

I can personally recommend *100 Perks of Having Cancer plus 100 Health Tips For Surviving It* http://www.amazon.com/100-Perks-Having-Cancer-Surviving-ebook/dp/B00ESFZ1BG by Florence Strang and Susan Gonzalez, mentioned previously. Each of Florence's perks, which are as uplifting as they are amusing, is accompanied by a health tip from Susan, a nurse and nutrition expert. Florence also gave a *TED talk* https://www.youtube.com/ watch?v=ZUhQoeatU8Y on how the book came about.

Finding Humor Through Cancer. http://www.huffingtonpost.com/ kate-matthews/breast-cancer-awareness_b_2204593.html?ir= Australia An interview with cartoonist Kate Matthews about her breast cancer experiences and her inspiration for her book of cartoons *The Little Pink Book of (mostly) Cancer Cartoons (in color!) http://www.amazon.com/Little-mostly-Cancer-Cartoons-color/ dp/0985789417*

Comedian Tg Notaro jokes about her bilateral mastectomy on this *YouTube* video. https://www.youtube.com/watch?v= SW3i9cU96OU

One free resource I found was a short book *How to Keep On Laughing—A Guide to Coping Humor.* http://www.harthosp.org/ por-tals/1/images/20/keeponlaughing.pdf This book was written by 12 women, of various ages and stages of breast cancer, who were part of an online support program run by the Hartford Hospital in Connecticut, USA.

Acknowledgments

I'd like to thank the wonderful women I mentioned in my Introduction, who so generously shared their experiences and emotions with me – Kay, Katie, Jan, Yvonne, Rochelle and Kath. I wish you all continuing health and happiness.

As always, I'm indebted to Pam Mariko and my partner Aaron for their suggestions and feedback.

I also sincerely thank Christine Cranney for her copyediting, my cover designer Judy Bullard for the great cover, and Maureen Cutajar for the formatting.

And last, but certainly not least, my grateful thanks to all the medical staff at Nambour Hospital and Oceania Oncology for looking after me so well, and Cancer Council Queensland and Breast Cancer Network Australia for their information and support.

Authors Love Reviews

Thank-you for buying this book and I hope you enjoyed it.

I would really appreciate it if you would post an honest review of this book on Amazon or whichever site you bought it from. Every review helps to give the book more exposure, helps other readers to decide if they want to buy the book and last but not least, helps me to sell more copies.

TALK TO ME!

I love chatting to readers, so please email me at robin@ alto-soft.com.au or connect with me on any of the sites below.

Website/blog storey-lines.com
Facebook www.facebook.com/RobinStoreywriter
Twitter twitter.com/RobinStorey1
Pinterest pinterest.com/robinstorey
LinkedIn www.linkedin.com/in/robinstoreyauthor
Instagram instagram.com/robinstorey55/
YouTube www.youtube.com/user/RobinStoreyAuthor
Goodreads www.goodreads.com/author/show/7057008.Robin_Storey

Other Books By Robin Storey

For books in the Noir Nights crime/suspense series and Robin's stand-alone novels, please visit Storey-Lines http://storey-lines.com or find Robin Storey on Amazon or Ingram Spark.

Made in the USA
Las Vegas, NV
08 December 2020